Certified Coding Associate (CCA) Exam Preparation

Seventh Edition

Rachael Gagner D'Andrea
MS, RHIA, CDIP, CHTS-TR, CPHQ
Editor

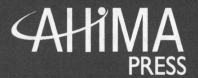

AHIMA PRESS

ISBN: 978-1-58426-703-4

AHIMA Product No.: AC400319

AHIMA Staff:

Chelsea Brotherton, Assistant Editor

Megan Grennan, Managing Editor

James Pinnick, Director of Publications

Cover image: © exdez iStock

For more information, including updates, about AHIMA Press publications, visit http://www.ahima .org/education/press.

American Health Information Management Association

233 North Michigan Avenue, 21st Floor

Chicago, Illinois 60601-5809

ahima.org

Contents

Practice Questions

Practice Exams

Answer Key

References

Online Assessments

Practice Questions with Answers
Practice Exam 1 with Answers
Practice Exam 2 with Answers

About the Editor

Rachael Gagner D'Andrea, MS, RHIA, CDIP, CHTS-TR, CPHQ, is a Consultant and Instructor for the State of CT and Lecturer for the State of FL college systems. She is Past President of the Connecticut Health Information Management Association (CtHIMA) and an editor and technical reviewer for multiple publications for AHIMA Press and author for Elsevier.

With over 30 years' experience in health information management (HIM), her career has encompassed several domains, including acute care, quality improvement, home health, software marketing and development, and education. She is a past director for CtHIMA, previous member of AHIMA's Clinical Practice Council, and contributor to Agency for Healthcare Research and Quality's ICD-10-CM/PCS transition workgroup. She has lectured extensively on coding, diagnosis-related groups, reimbursement and data quality issues throughout the United States and internationally.

As an educator—both nationally and internationally—and an active committee member of AHIMA's Assembly on Education, Envision, National Association for Healthcare Quality, and ICD-10 Expert, Ms. D'Andrea continues to advance her knowledge in our dynamic profession with the observation that we in HIM are never finished learning. She promotes and supports this direction for all HIM professionals.

Ms. D'Andrea has her master's degree in health informatics and information management from the College of St. Scholastica.

Acknowledgments

The editor and AHIMA Press would like to thank Gloria Anderson, MEd, RHIA, CCS for serving as technical reviewer of this edition.

About the CCA Examination

The CCA exam consists of 100 multiple choice questions. Candidates have two hours to complete the exam. The Commission on Certification for Health Informatics and Information Management (CCHIIM) manages and sets the strategic direction for the certifications. Pearson Vue is the exclusive provider of AHIMA certification exams. To see sample questions and images of the new exam format, visit http://www.ahima.org/certification/CCA.

Detailed information about the CCA exam and academic eligibility requirements can be found at www.ahima.org/certification.

The National Commission for Certifying Agencies (NCCA) has granted accreditation to AHIMA's CCA certification program for demonstrating compliance with the NCCA Standards for the Accreditation of Certification Programs. NCCA is the accrediting body of the Institute for Credentialing Excellence (formerly the National Organization for Competency Assurance).

The NCCA Standards were created in 1977 and updated in 2014 to ensure certification programs adhere to modern standards of practice for the certification industry. AHIMA joins an elite group of more than 100 organizations representing more than 200 programs that have received and maintained NCCA accreditation. More information on the NCCA is available online at http://www.credentialingexcellence.org/ncca.

Exam Competency Statements

A certification exam is based on an explicit set of competencies. These competencies have been determined through a job analysis study of practitioners. The competencies are subdivided into domains and tasks, as listed here. The exam tests only content pertaining to these competencies. Each domain is allocated a predefined number of questions at specific cognitive levels to make up the exam.

Domain 1: Clinical Classification Systems (30–34% of Exam)

1. Interpret healthcare data for code assignment
2. Incorporate clinical vocabularies and terminologies used in health information systems
3. Abstract pertinent information from medical records
4. Consult reference materials to facilitate code assignment
5. Apply inpatient coding guidelines
6. Apply outpatient coding guidelines
7. Apply physician coding guidelines
8. Assign inpatient codes
9. Assign outpatient codes
10. Assign physician codes
11. Sequence codes according to healthcare setting

Domain 2: Reimbursement Methodologies (21–25% of Exam)

1. Sequence codes for optimal reimbursement
2. Link diagnoses and CPT codes according to payer specific guidelines
3. Assign correct diagnosis-related group (DRG)

4. Assign correct ambulatory payment classification (APC)
5. Evaluate NCCI (National Correct Coding Initiative) edits
6. Reconcile NCCI edits
7. Validate medical necessity using LCDs (local coverage determinations) and NCDs (national coverage determinations)
8. Submit claim forms
9. Communicate with financial departments
10. Evaluate claim denials
11. Respond to claim denials
12. Resubmit denied claim to the payer source
13. Communicate with the physician to clarify documentation

Domain 3: Health Records and Data Content (13–17% of Exam)

1. Retrieve medical records
2. Assemble medical records according to healthcare setting
3. Analyze medical records quantitatively for completeness
4. Analyze medical records qualitatively for deficiencies
5. Perform data abstraction
6. Request patient-specific documentation from other sources (for example, ancillary departments, physician's office)
7. Retrieve patient information from master patient index
8. Educate providers in regard to health data standards
9. Generate reports for data analysis

Domain 4: Compliance (12–16% of Exam)

1. Identify discrepancies between coded data and supporting documentation
2. Validate that codes assigned by provider or electronic systems are supported by proper documentation
3. Perform ethical coding
4. Clarify documentation through physician query
5. Research latest coding changes
6. Implement latest coding changes
7. Update fee/charge ticket based on latest coding changes
8. Educate providers on compliant coding
9. Assist in preparing the organization for external audits

Domain 5: Information Technologies (6–10% of Exam)

1. Navigate throughout the electronic health record (EHR)
2. Utilize encoding and grouping software
3. Utilize practice management and HIM systems
4. Utilize computer-assisted coding (CAC) software that automatically assigns codes based on electronic text
5. Validate the codes assigned by CAC software

Domain 6: Confidentiality and Privacy (6–10% of Exam)

1. Ensure patient confidentiality
2. Educate healthcare staff on privacy and confidentiality issues
3. Recognize and report privacy issues/violations
4. Maintain a secure work environment
5. Utilize pass codes
6. Access only minimal necessary documents/information
7. Release patient-specific data to authorized individuals
8. Protect electronic documents through encryption
9. Transfer electronic documents through secure sites
10. Retain confidential records appropriately
11. Destroy confidential records appropriately

How to Use This Book and Online Assessment

The CCA practice questions and practice exams in this book and on the accompanying online assessments test knowledge of content pertaining to the CCA competencies published by AHIMA. The 400 multiple choice questions in this book and online assessments are presented in a similar format to those that might be found on the CCA exam.

This book contains 200 multiple choice practice questions and two multiple choice practice exams (with 100 questions each). Because each question is identified with one of the six CCA domains, you will be able to determine whether you need knowledge or skill building in particular areas of the exam. Each question provides an answer rationale and reference. Pursuing the sources of these references will help build your knowledge and skills.

To most effectively use this book, work through all the practice questions first. This will help identify areas in which you may need further preparation. After going through the practice questions, take one of the practice exams. Again, for the questions that you answer incorrectly, refresh your knowledge by reading the associated references. Continue in the same manner with the second practice exam.

The online assessments present the same 200 practice questions and two timed practice exams printed in the book. These exams can be run in practice mode—which allows you to work at your own pace—or exam simulation mode—which simulates the two-hour, timed exam experience. You may retake the practice questions and exams as many times as you like. The practice questions and simulated practice exams online can be set to be presented in random order, or you may choose to go through the questions in sequential order by domain. You may also choose to practice or test your skills on specific domains. For example, if you would like to build your skills in domain 2, you may choose only domain 2 questions for a given practice session.

Test Taking Tips

The best way to prepare for the CCA certification exam is to study the material you have learned over the course of your health information management educational program. Because it is difficult to remember everything you have learned over the course of the program, it is important to review the information. This is best done using this exam preparation guide and the tips found above in How to Use This Book and Online Assessment. Carefully review the information in the Commission on Certification for Health Informatics and Information Management Candidate Guide (http://www.ahima.org/ /media/AHIMA/Files/Certification/Candidate_Guide.ashx). You will want to prepare yourself mentally, physically, and emotionally to succeed.

Other tips for studying:
- Be sure to get enough sleep.
- Eat a healthy, well balanced diet.
- Stay hydrated.
- Take breaks.
- Get some exercise.
- Do not try to memorize everything; work at understanding.
- Use tricks to remember the material, like using an acronym or other type of word or visual association.
- Try to eliminate other stressors, if possible.
- Take a practice exam in the two hour time frame you will have for the exam.
- If you do not know where the testing center is located, visit it before the day of the exam. This will help you avoid getting lost or being late for your exam.

Exam Day Tips

- Get enough sleep in the days leading up to the exam.
- Wear clothes that you are comfortable in and dress in layers so that you can remove or add a sweater based on the temperature of the room.
- Eat a healthy breakfast and give yourself enough time to get ready to leave so you are not rushed.
- Arrive at the testing center 30 minutes prior to your exam time with your required identification.
- You will have two hours to complete the exam. Do not obsess over the clock in the room, but do budget your time. This should allow you to answer each question and review any questions you may want to revisit. Time management will be an important part of taking the exam.
- Be sure to read each question carefully. Do not automatically assume you know the answer to a question without first reading the entire question and each answer choice carefully. After reviewing each answer, choose the best answer.
- Skip questions that you do not know the answer to or that are difficult and come back to them. You may find something in another question that helps you to recall information you need to answer a question you skipped. Be sure to manage your time well while you do this.
- Be sure to answer every test question. A guess is better than not taking the opportunity to answer a question. But, do so after carefully reviewing the question and the possible answers. After eliminating answers you know are incorrect, make the best selection. A true guess will give you a one-in-four chance of getting a question correct.
- Remember to relax as much as possible and BREATHE. You can do this!

PRACTICE QUESTIONS

Domain 1 *Clinical Classification Systems*

1. Identify the diagnosis code(s) for carcinoma in situ of vocal cord.

   a. D02.0

   b. C32.0

   c. D49.1

   d. D14.1

2. Identify the diagnosis code(s) for melanoma of skin of right shoulder.

   a. D03.61, C43.61

   b. C43.61

   c. C43.60

   d. D03.61

3. Which of the following organizations is responsible for updating the procedure classification of ICD-10-PCS?

   a. Centers for Disease Control (CDC)

   b. Centers for Medicare and Medicaid Services (CMS)

   c. National Center for Health Statistics (NCHS)

   d. World Health Organization (WHO)

4. "Code, if applicable, on causal condition first," note indicates that this code may be assigned as a first listed or principal diagnosis when:

   a. the causal condition is a symptom code

   b. the code for the condition is unrelated to the causal condition

   c. the causal condition is unknown or not applicable

   d. the code appears in italicized font

5. Which character in an ICD-10-CM diagnosis code provides information regarding encounter of care?

   a. Fourth

   b. Fifth

   c. Sixth

   d. Seventh

6. What does the fourth character of an ICD-10-CM diagnosis code capture?

   a. Anatomic site

   b. Severity

   c. Etiology

   d. Supplemental information

7. ICD-10-CM codes must be a minimum length of how many characters?

    a. Three

    b. Five

    c. Six

    d. Seven

8. Notes appearing under a 3-character code apply to which of the following?

    a. Only to category codes that are exactly three-characters long

    b. To all codes within that category

    c. Only to one specific code

    d. To all codes within that chapter

9. Which volume of ICD-10-CM contains the Tabular and Alphabetic Index of procedures?

    a. Volume 1

    b. Volume 2

    c. Volume 3

    d. None of the above

10. An exception to the Excludes 1 definition is the circumstance when the two conditions _____.

    a. Are unrelated to each other

    b. Are related to each other

    c. Will not be assigned as the principal diagnosis

    d. Are injuries with external cause codes

11. Identify the correct diagnosis code(s) for adenoma of left adrenal cortex with Conn's syndrome.

    a. D35.02, E26.01

    b. D35.02

    c. E26.01

    d. E26.01, D35.7

12. Which of the following is a standard terminology used to code medical procedures and services?

    a. CPT

    b. HCPCS

    c. ICD-10-PCS

    d. SNOMED CT

13. Identify the appropriate ICD-10-CM diagnosis code for right cerebral contusion with 15-minute loss of consciousness, initial encounter for care.

    a. T14.8

    b. S06.371A

    c. S06.311A

    d. S06.310A

14. If a patient has an excision of a malignant lesion of the skin, the CPT code is determined by the body area from which the excision occurs and which of the following?

    a. Length of the lesion as described in the pathology report

    b. Dimension of the specimen submitted as described in the pathology report

    c. Width times the length of the lesion as described in the operative report

    d. Diameter of the lesion as well as the most narrow margins required to adequately excise the lesion described in the operative report

15. According to CPT, a repair of a laceration that includes retention sutures would be considered what type of closure?

    a. Simple

    b. Intermediate

    c. Complex

    d. Not specified

16. A patient is admitted with spotting. She had been treated two weeks previously for a miscarriage with sepsis. The sepsis had resolved, and she is afebrile at this time. She is treated with an aspiration dilation and curettage and products of conception are found. Which of the following should be the principal diagnosis?

    a. Miscarriage

    b. Complications of spontaneous abortion with sepsis

    c. Sepsis

    d. Spontaneous abortion with sepsis

17. An 80-year-old female is admitted with fever, lethargy, hypotension, tachycardia, oliguria, and elevated WBC. The patient has more than 100,000 organisms of *Escherichia coli* per cc of urine. The attending physician documents "urosepsis." How should the coder proceed to code this case?

    a. Code sepsis as the principal diagnosis with urinary tract infection due to *E. coli* as secondary diagnosis.

    b. Code urinary tract infection with sepsis as the principal diagnosis.

    c. Query the physician to determine if the patient has sepsis due to the symptomatology.

    d. Query the physician to determine if the patient has septic shock so that this may be used as the principal diagnosis.

18. A 65-year-old patient, with a history of lung cancer, is admitted to a healthcare facility with ataxia and syncope and a fractured arm as a result of falling. The patient undergoes a closed reduction of the fracture in the emergency department and undergoes a complete workup for metastatic carcinoma of the brain. The patient is found to have metastatic carcinoma of the lung to the brain and undergoes radiation therapy to the brain. Which of the following would be the principal diagnosis in this case?

    a. Ataxia

    b. Fractured arm

    c. Metastatic carcinoma of the brain

    d. Carcinoma of the lung

19. A patient was admitted for abdominal pain with diarrhea and was diagnosed with infectious gastroenteritis. The patient also has angina and chronic obstructive pulmonary disease. Which of the following would be the correct coding and sequencing for this case?

    a. Abdominal pain; infectious gastroenteritis; chronic obstructive pulmonary disease; angina

    b. Infectious gastroenteritis; chronic obstructive pulmonary disease; angina

    c. Gastroenteritis; abdominal pain; angina

    d. Gastroenteritis; abdominal pain; diarrhea; chronic obstructive pulmonary disease; angina

20. Patient has been diagnosed with acute depression, sleep-related teeth grinding and psychogenic dysmenorrhea. The appropriate code assignment is:

    a. F32.8, F45.8

    b. F32.9, F45.8

    c. F32.9, F45.8, G47.63

    d. F32.9, G47.53

21. A patient is admitted with abdominal pain. The physician documents the discharge diagnosis as pancreatitis versus noncalculus cholecystitis. Both diagnoses are equally treated. The correct coding and sequencing for this case would be:

    a. Sequence either the pancreatitis or noncalculus cholecystitis as principal diagnosis

    b. Pancreatitis; noncalculus cholecystitis; abdominal pain

    c. Noncalculus cholecystitis; pancreatitis; abdominal pain

    d. Abdominal pain; pancreatitis; noncalculus cholecystitis

22. According to the UHDDS, which of the following is the definition of "other diagnoses"?

    a. Is recorded in the patient record

    b. Is documented by the attending physician

    c. Receives clinical evaluation or therapeutic treatment or diagnostic procedures or extends the length of stay or increases nursing care and monitoring

    d. Is documented by at least two physicians and the nursing staff

23. A 7-year-old patient was admitted to the emergency department for treatment of shortness of breath. The patient is given epinephrine and nebulizer treatments. The shortness of breath and wheezing are unabated following treatment. What diagnosis should be suspected?

    a. Acute bronchitis

    b. Acute bronchitis with chronic obstructive pulmonary disease

    c. Asthma with status asthmaticus

    d. Chronic obstructive asthma

24. A patient is seen in the emergency department for chest pain. After evaluation of the patient it is suspected that the patient may have gastroesophageal reflux disease (GERD). The final diagnosis was "chest pain versus GERD." The correct ICD-10-CM code is:

    a. Z03.89 Encounter for observation for other suspected diseases and conditions ruled out

    b. R10.11 Right upper quadrant abdominal pain

    c. K21.9 Gastro-esophageal reflux disease

    d. R07.9 Chest pain, unspecified

25. A skin lesion is removed from a patient's cheek in the dermatologist's office. The dermatologist documents "skin lesion" in the health record. Before billing, the pathology report returns with a diagnosis of basal cell carcinoma. Which of the following actions should the coding professional do for claim submission?

    a. Code skin lesion

    b. Code benign skin lesion

    c. Code basal cell carcinoma

    d. Query the dermatologist

26. An epidural was given during labor. Subsequently, it was determined that the patient would require a C-section for cephalopelvic disproportion because of obstructed labor. Assign the correct ICD-10-CM diagnostic and CPT anesthesia codes. (Modifiers are not used in this example.)

    a. O65.4, 64479

    b. O65.4, O33.0, 01961

    c. O65.4, 01967, 01968

    d. O65.4, O33.9, 01996

27. Which of the following purpose and use goals does *not* apply to ICD-10-PCS?

    a. Improved accuracy and efficiency of coding

    b. Reduced training effort

    c. Improved communication with physicians

    d. Improved collection of data about nursing care

28. When present, conditions that are not an integral part of the disease process

    a. should never be coded

    b. should prompt a physician query

    c. are always coded

    d. should be assigned from the signs and symptoms codes

29. To help clarify terms that currently have overlapping meaning, ICD-10-PCS has defined root operations. What is an example of the root operation of Excision?

    a. Partial nephrectomy

    b. Total nephrectomy

    c. Total lobectomy

    d. Total mastectomy

30. The assignment of a diagnosis code is based on _____.

    a. The coder's assessment of the health record

    b. The provider's statement that the patient has a particular condition

    c. Clinical criteria used by the provider to establish the diagnosis

    d. Its inclusion in the discharge summary

31. A patient was discharged with the following diagnoses: "Cerebral artery occlusion, hemiparesis, and hypertension. The aphasia resolved before the patient was discharged." Which of the following code assignments would be appropriate for this case?

G81.90	Hemiparesis affecting unspecified side
G81.91	Hemiparesis affecting right dominant side
G81.92	Hemiparesis affecting left dominant side
G81.94	Hemiparesis affecting left nondominant side
I66.9	Cerebral artery occlusion unspecified, without mention of cerebral infarction
I63.50	Cerebral artery occlusion unspecified with cerebral infarction
I10	Hypertension
I50.9	Congestive heart failure
R47.01	Aphasia

a. I63.50, G81.94, R47.01, I10

b. I66.9, G81.90, R47.01, I10

c. I66.9, G81.91, I10

d. I66.9, G81.92, R47.01, I10

32. A patient is admitted to the hospital with shortness of breath and congestive heart failure. The patient subsequently develops respiratory failure. The patient undergoes intubation with ventilator management. Which of the following would be the correct sequencing and coding of this case?

a. Congestive heart failure, respiratory failure, ventilator management

b. Respiratory failure, intubation, ventilator management

c. Respiratory failure, congestive heart failure, intubation, ventilator management

d. Shortness of breath, congestive heart failure, respiratory failure, ventilator management

33. A physician correctly prescribes Coumadin. The patient takes the Coumadin as prescribed but develops hematuria as a result of taking the medication. Which of the following is the correct way to code this case?

a. Poisoning due to Coumadin

b. Unspecified adverse reaction to Coumadin

c. Hematuria; poisoning due to Coumadin

d. Hematuria; adverse reaction to Coumadin

34. A patient is admitted for chest pain with cardiac dysrhythmia to Hospital A. The patient is found to have an acute ST elevation (STEMI) inferior myocardial infarction with atrial fibrillation. After the atrial fibrillation was controlled and the patient was stabilized, the patient was transferred to Hospital B for a CABG X3. Coumadin therapy and monitoring for the atrial fibrillation continued at Hospital B. Using the codes listed here, what are the appropriate ICD-10-CM codes and sequencing for both hospitalizations?

I21.09	Myocardial infarction of anterior wall, initial
I21.19	Myocardial infarction of inferior wall, initial
I22.0	Myocardial infarction of anterolateral wall, subsequent
I22.1	Myocardial infarction of inferior wall, subsequent
I48.0	Paroxysmal atrial fibrillation
I48.2	Chronic atrial fibrillation
I48.91	Unspecified atrial fibrillation
R07.9	Chest pain, unspecified
021209W	Aortocoronary bypass, Three Sites from Aorta with Autologous Venous Tissue, Open Approach

   a. Hospital A: I48.91, R07.9, I21.19; Hospital B: I22.1, I48.91, 021209W
   b. Hospital A: I21.09, I48.0; Hospital B: I22.0, I48.2, 021209W
   c. Hospital A: I21.19, I48.91; Hospital B: I21.19, I48.91, 021209W
   d. Hospital A: I21.19, I48.91; Hospital B: I22.1, I48.91, 021209W

35. A patient is admitted to the hospital with abdominal pain. The principal diagnosis is cholecystitis. The patient also has a history of hypertension and diabetes. In the DRG prospective payment system, which of the following would determine the MDC assignment for this patient?

   a. Abdominal pain
   b. Cholecystitis
   c. Hypertension
   d. Diabetes

36. A patient was admitted to the hospital with symptoms of a stroke and secondary diagnoses of COPD and hypertension. The patient was subsequently discharged from the hospital with a principal diagnosis of cerebral vascular accident and secondary diagnoses of catheter-associated urinary tract infection, COPD, and hypertension. Which of the following diagnoses should *not* be tagged as POA?

   a. Catheter-associated urinary tract infection
   b. Cerebral vascular accident
   c. COPD
   d. Hypertension

37. Which of the following is a condition that arises during hospitalization?

   a. Case mix
   b. Complication
   c. Comorbidity
   d. Principal diagnosis

38. A 65-year-old female was admitted to the hospital. She was diagnosed with sepsis secondary to *Staphylococcus aureus* and abdominal pain secondary to diverticulitis of the colon. What is the correct code assignment?

    a. A41.89, K57.92, R10.9

    b. A41.01, K57.92

    c. A41.89, K57.92, A49.01

    d. A41.9, K57.92

39. Patient had carcinoma of the anterior bladder wall fulgurated three years ago. The patient returns yearly for a cystoscopy to recheck for bladder tumor. Patient is currently admitted for a routine check. A small recurring malignancy is found and fulgurated during the cystoscopy procedure. Which is the correct code assignment?

    a. C67.3, Z85.51, 0T5B8ZZ, 0TJB8ZZ

    b. C79.11, 0T5B8ZZ

    c. C67.3, 0T5B8ZZ

    d. C79.11, C67.3, 0T5B8ZZ

40. For the body mass index (BMI), depth of non-pressure chronic ulcers, pressure ulcer stage, coma scale, and NIH stroke scale (NIHSS) codes, code assignment may be based on _____.

    a. Medical record documentation from clinicians who are not the patient's provider (i.e., physician or other qualified healthcare practitioner legally accountable for establishing the patient's diagnosis)

    b. Only the attending physician's documentation

    c. Consulting physicians' report

    d. The history and physical report

41. These codes are used to assign a diagnosis to a patient who is seeking health services but is not necessarily sick.

    a. C codes

    b. E codes

    c. M codes

    d. Z codes

42. Patient was admitted through the emergency department following a fall from a ladder while painting an interior bathroom in his farmhouse. He had contusions of the scalp and face and a displaced open fracture of the anterior wall of the right acetabulum. The fracture site was excisionally debrided and the fracture was reduced by open procedure with an internal fixation device inserted. Which is the correct code assignment?

    a. S32.411A, W11XXA, Y92.012, 0QS404Z, 0QB40ZZ

    b. S32.411B, S00.03XA, S00.83XA, W11.XXXA, Y92.012, Y93.E9, Y99.8, 0QS404Z, 0QB40ZZ

    c. S32.414A, W11.XXA, Y93.E9, Y99.8, 0QS304Z, 0QB50ZZ

    d. S32.411B, W11.XXA, Y92.012, Y93.E9, 0QS404Z, 0QB50ZZ

43. Assign the correct CPT code for the following procedure: Reposition of the pacemaker electrode.

    a. 33226

    b. 33243

    c. 33217

    d. 33215

44. Assign the correct CPT code for the following: A 58-year-old male was seen in the outpatient surgical center for an extensive destruction of penile lesion by laser.

    a. 54065

    b. 54060

    c. 54057

    d. 54050

45. Patient returns during a 90-day postoperative period from a ventral hernia repair, now complaining of eye pain. What modifier would a physician setting use with the Evaluation and Management code?

    a. −79, Unrelated procedure or service by the same physician during the postoperative period

    b. −25, Significant, separately identifiable evaluation and management service by the same physician on the same day of the procedure or other service

    c. −21, Prolonged evaluation and management services

    d. −24, Unrelated evaluation and management service by the same physician during a postoperative period

46. A patient is admitted to an acute-care hospital for alcohol abuse and uncomplicated alcohol withdrawal syndrome due to chronic alcoholism. His blood alcohol level on admission was 10 mg/100 mL.

    a. F10.230, F10.10, Y90.0

    b. F10.230

    c. F10.10, Y90.0

    d. F10.230, Y90.0

47. A 45-year-old female is admitted for blood loss anemia due to dysfunctional uterine bleeding.

    a. D50.0, N93.8

    b. D62, N93.8

    c. N93.8, D50.0

    d. D50.0, D25.9

48. Patient admitted with left senile cortical cataract, diabetes mellitus, and extracapsular cataract extraction with simultaneous insertion of synthetic intraocular lens, via percutaneous approach.

    a. H25.012, E11.36, 08DK3ZZ, 08RK3JZ

    b. E11.9, H25.012

    c. E11.9, H25.092

    d. H25.012, E11.9, 08RK3JZ

49. A patient is admitted with acute exacerbation of COPD, chronic renal failure, and hypertension.

    a. J44.1, J44.9, I12.9, N18.9
    b. J44.1, N18.9, I10
    c. J44.9, N18.9, I10
    d. J44.1, I12.9, N18.9

50. Code only a confirmed diagnosis of Zika virus (A92.5, Zika virus disease) as documented by the provider. In this context, "confirmation" _____.

    a. Does not require documentation of the type of test performed; the physician's diagnostic statement that the condition is confirmed is sufficient
    b. Requires the documentation of the type of test in addition to the physician's diagnostic statement
    c. Must be provided by the laboratory findings report
    d. Requires that the Public Health Agency be contacted

51. The patient was admitted to the outpatient department and had a bronchoscopy with bronchial brushings performed.

    a. 31622, 31640
    b. 31622, 31623
    c. 31623
    d. 31625

52. Identify the two-digit modifier that may be reported to indicate a physician performed the postoperative management of a patient, but another physician performed the surgical procedure.

    a. −22
    b. −54
    c. −32
    d. −55

53. What is the correct CPT code assignment for destruction of internal hemorrhoids with use of infrared coagulation?

    a. 46255
    b. 46930
    c. 46260
    d. 46945

54. An encoder that takes a coder through a series of questions and choices is called a(n):

    a. Automated codebook
    b. Automated code assignment
    c. Logic-based encoder
    d. Decision support database

55. The patient was admitted with major depression current episode severe, recurrent. What is the correct ICD-10-CM diagnosis code assignment for this condition?

    a. F33.2

    b. F33.40

    c. F32.9

    d. F31.81

56. A 35-year-old male was admitted with heartburn that has not improved with over-the-counter medications. An esophagoscopy and closed esophageal biopsy at the upper esophagus was performed. The physician documented esophageal reflux with esophagitis as the final diagnosis based on pathological examination. Identify the correct diagnosis and procedure codes.

    a. K23, 0DJ07ZZ

    b. K20.9, 0DB58ZX

    c. K21.0, 0DB18ZX

    d. K21.9, 0DB18ZX

57. Patient with flank pain was admitted and found to have a calculus of the kidney. A ureteroscopy with placement of bilateral ureteral stents was performed to expand the lumen so the stone could pass naturally. Assign the correct ICD-10-CM/PCS diagnosis and procedure codes.

    a. N20.0, N23, 0T788DZ

    b. N23, N20.0, 0TC68ZZ, 0TC78ZZ

    c. N20.0, 0T768DZ, 0T778DZ

    d. N20.0, 0T788DZ

58. A female patient is admitted for stress incontinence. A urethral suspension to reposition the urethra via open approach is performed. Assign the correct ICD-10-CM diagnosis and/or procedure codes.

    a. N39.3, 0TJB8ZZ

    b. N23, 0TSD0ZZ

    c. N39.3, 0TSD0ZZ

    d. R32, 0TSD4ZZ

59. Reference codes 49491 through 49525 for inguinal hernia repair. Patient is 47 years old. What is the correct code for an initial inguinal herniorrhaphy for incarcerated hernia?

    a. 49496

    b. 49501

    c. 49507

    d. 49521

60. If the documentation in a medical record does not indicate the type of diabetes but does indicate that the patient uses insulin, _____.

    a. Code E10, Type 1 diabetes mellitus, should be assigned.

    b. Code E11, Type 2 diabetes mellitus, should be assigned.

    c. Query the endocrinologist or attending physician.

    d. Check the physician orders or medical order record for additional information.

61. What is the correct CPT code assignment for hysteroscopy with lysis of intrauterine adhesions?

    a. 58555, 58559

    b. 58559

    c. 58559, 58740

    d. 58555, 58559, 58740

62. The physician performs an exploratory laparotomy with bilateral salpingo-oophorectomy. What is the correct CPT code assignment for this procedure?

    a. 49000, 58940, 58700

    b. 58940, 58720–50

    c. 49000, 58720

    d. 58720

63. Identify the CPT code for a 42-year-old diagnosed with ESRD who requires home dialysis for the month of April.

    a. 90965

    b. 90964

    c. 90966

    d. 90970

64. The patient presented to the physical therapy department and received 30 minutes of water aerobics therapeutic exercise with the therapist for treatment of arthritis. What is the appropriate treatment code(s) or modifier for a Medicare patient on a physical therapy plan of care in an outpatient setting?

    a. 97113

    b. 97113–50

    c. 97113, 97113

    d. 97110

Domain 2 *Reimbursement Methodologies*

65. Given the following information, which of the following statements is correct?

	MCD	Type	MS-DRG Title	Weight	Discharges	Geometric Mean	Arithmetic Mean
191	04	MED	Chronic obstructive pulmonary disease w CC	0.9757	10	4.1	5.0
192	04	MED	Chronic obstructive pulmonary disease w/o CC/MCC	0.7254	20	3.3	4.0
193	04	MED	Simple pneumonia & pleurisy w MCC	1.4327	10	5.4	6.7
194	04	MED	Simple pneumonia & pleurisy w CC	1.0056	20	4.4	5.3
195	04	MED	Simple pneumonia & pleurisy w/o CC/MCC	0.7316	10	3.5	4.1

    a. In each MS-DRG the geometric mean is lower than the arithmetic mean.

    b. In each MS-DRG the arithmetic mean is lower than the geometric mean.

    c. The higher the number of patients in each MS-DRG, the greater the geometric mean for that MS-DRG.

    d. The geometric means are lower in MS-DRGs that are associated with a CC or MCC.

66. If another status T procedure were performed, how much would the facility receive for the second status T procedure?

Billing Number	Status Indicator	CPT/HCPCS	APC
998323	V	99285–25	0612
998324	T	25500	0044
998325	X	72050	0261
998326	S	72128	0283
998327	S	70450	0283

    a. 0%

    b. 50%

    c. 75%

    d. 100%

67. Medical necessity for inpatient services does not always include:

    a. LCDs

    b. Related monetary benefits to payers

    c. Uniform written procedures for appeals

    d. Concurrent review

68. Which of the following types of hospitals are excluded from the Medicare inpatient prospective payment system?

    a. Children's

    b. Rural

    c. State supported

    d. Tertiary

69. Diagnosis-related groups are organized into:

    a. Case-mix classifications

    b. Geographic practice cost indices

    c. Major diagnostic categories

    d. Resource-based relative values

70. The Medicare program pays for health care services Social Security benefits for those age 65 and older, permanently disabled people and those with:

    a. End stage renal disease

    b. Military experience

    c. Medicaid

    d. Skilled nursing services

71. Which of the following is *not* reimbursed according to the Medicare outpatient prospective payment system?

    a. CMHC partial hospitalization services

    b. Critical access hospitals

    c. Hospital outpatient departments

    d. Vaccines provided by CORFs

72. Fee schedules are updated by third-party payers:

    a. Annually

    b. Monthly

    c. Semiannually

    d. Weekly

73. Which of the following would a health record technician use to perform the billing function for a physician's office?

    a. CMS-1500

    b. UB-04

    c. UB-92

    d. CMS 1450

74. When a provider accepts assignment, this means the:

    a. Patient authorizes payment to be made directly to the provider

    b. Provider agrees to accept as payment in full the allowed charge from the fee schedule

    c. Balance billing is allowed on patient accounts, but at a limited rate

    d. Participating provider receives a fee-for-service reimbursement

75. A coding audit shows that an inpatient coder is using multiple codes that describe the individual components of a procedure rather than using a single code that describes all the steps of the procedure performed. Which of the following should be done in this case?

    a. Require all coders to implement this practice

    b. Report the practice to the OIG

    c. Counsel the coder and stop the practice immediately

    d. Put the coder on unpaid leave of absence

76. Prospective payment systems were developed by the federal government to:

    a. Increase healthcare access

    b. Manage Medicare and Medicaid costs

    c. Implement managed care programs

    d. Eliminate fee-for-service programs

77. Given NCCI edits, if the placement of a catheter is billed along with the performance of an infusion procedure for the same date of service for an outpatient beneficiary, Medicare will pay for:

    a. The placement of the catheter

    b. The placement of the catheter and the infusion procedure

    c. The infusion procedure

    d. Neither the placement of the catheter nor the infusion procedure

78. The goal of coding compliance programs is to reduce:

    a. Liability in regards to fraud and abuse

    b. Delays in claims processing

    c. Billing errors

    d. Inaccurate code assignments

79. Which of the following actions would be best to determine whether present on admission (POA) indicators for the conditions selected by CMS are having a negative impact on the hospital's Medicare reimbursement?

    a. Identify all records for a period having these indicators for these conditions and determine if these conditions are the only secondary diagnoses present on the claim that will lead to higher payment.

    b. Identify all records for a period that have these indicators for these conditions.

    c. Identify all records for a period that have these indicators for these conditions and determine whether or not additional documentation can be submitted to Medicare to increase reimbursement.

    d. Take a random sample of records for a period of time for records having these indicators for these conditions and extrapolate the negative impact on Medicare reimbursement.

80. From the information provided, how many APCs would this patient have?

Billing Number	Status Indicator	CPT/HCPCS	APC
998323	V	99285–25	0612
998324	T	25500	0044
998325	X	72050	0261
998326	S	72128	0283
998327	S	70450	0283

   a. 1

   b. 4

   c. 5

   d. 3

81. If a patient's total outpatient bill is $500, and the patient's healthcare insurance plan pays 80% of the allowable charges, what is the amount owed by the patient?

   a. $10

   b. $40

   c. $100

   d. $400

82. In a managed fee-for-service arrangement, which of the following would be used as a cost-control process for inpatient surgical services?

   a. Prospectively precertify the necessity of inpatient services

   b. Determine what services can be bundled

   c. Pay only 80% of the inpatient bill

   d. Require the patient to pay 20% of the inpatient bill

83. The sum of a hospital's total relative DRG weights for a year was 15,192 and the hospital had 10,471 total discharges for the year. Given this information, what would be the hospital's case-mix index for that year?

   a. 0.689

   b. 1.59

   c. 1.45×100

   d. 1.45

84. In processing a bill under the Medicare outpatient prospective payment system (OPPS) in which a patient had three surgical procedures performed during the same operative session, which of the following would apply?

   a. Bundling of services

   b. Outlier adjustment

   c. Pass-through payment

   d. Discounting of procedures

85. The government sponsored supplemental medical insurance that covers physicians and surgeons services, emergency department, outpatient clinic, labs and physical therapy is:

    a. Medicaid

    b. Medicare Part B

    c. Medicare Part A

    d. Medicare Part D

86. A denial of a claim is possible for all of the following reasons *except*:

    a. Not meeting medical necessity

    b. Billing too many units of a specific service

    c. Unbundling

    d. Approved precertification

87. Promoting correct coding and control of inappropriate payments is the basis of NCCI claims processing edits that help identify claims not meeting medical necessity. The NCCI automated prepayment edits used by payers is based on all of the following *except*:

    a. Coding conventions defined in the CPT book

    b. National and local policies and coding edits

    c. Analysis of standard medical and surgical practice

    d. Clinical documentation in the discharge summary

88. The NCCI editing system used in processing OPPS claims is referred to as:

    a. Outpatient code editor (OCE)

    b. Outpatient national editor (ONE)

    c. Outpatient perspective payment editor (OPPE)

    d. Outpatient claims editor (OCE)

89. Denials of outpatient claims are often generated from all of the following edits *except*:

    a. NCCI (National Correct Coding Initiative)

    b. OCE (outpatient code editor)

    c. OCE (outpatient claims editor)

    d. National and local policies

90. Timely and correct reimbursement is dependent on:

    a. Adjudication

    b. Clean claims

    c. Remittance advice

    d. Actual charge

91. Solutions to address the problem of dirty claims include all of the following *except*:

    a. Submitting paper claims

    b. Submitting claims electronically

    c. Using electronic health record system that eliminates manual or duplicate entry of data

    d. Auditing claims' accuracy and compliance with edits prior to submitting

92. Which of the following is *not* an essential data element for a healthcare insurance claim?

    a. Revenue code

    b. Procedure code

    c. Provider name

    d. Procedure name

93. The next generation of consumer-directed healthcare will be driven by a design where copayments are set based on the value of the clinical services rather than the traditional practices that focus only on costs of clinical services. What new design will focus on both the benefit and cost?

    a. Value-based insurance design (VBID)

    b. Cost-based reimbursement (CBR)

    c. Pay for performance design (PPD)

    d. Prospective payment system (PPS)

94. Effective October 16, 2003, under the Administrative Simplification Compliance section of the Health Insurance Portability and Accountability Act of 1996 (HIPAA), all healthcare providers must electronically submit claims to Medicare. Which is the electronic format for hospital technical fees?

    a. 837I

    b. 837P

    c. UB-04

    d. 1500

95. The government sponsored program that provides expanded coverage of many health care services including HMO plans, PPO plans, special needs and Medical Savings accounts is:

    a. Medicare Advantage

    b. Medicare Part A

    c. Medicare Part B

    d. Medigap

96. When clean claims are submitted, they can be adjudicated in many ways through computer software automatically. Which statement is *not* one of the outcomes that can occur as part of auto-adjudication?

    a. Auto-pay

    b. Auto-suspend

    c. Auto-calculate

    d. Auto-deny

97. What system assigns each service a value representing the true resources involved in producing it, including the time and intensity of work, the expenses of practice, and the risk of malpractice?

    a. DRGs

    b. RVUs

    c. CPT

    d. SVR

98. What statement is *not* reflective of meeting medical necessity requirements?

    a. A service or supply provided for the diagnosis, treatment, cure, or relief of a health condition, illness, injury, or disease.

    b. A service or supply provided that is not experimental, investigational, or cosmetic in purpose.

    c. A service provided that is necessary for and appropriate to the diagnosis, treatment, cure, or relief of a health condition, illness, injury, disease, or its symptoms.

    d. A service provided solely for the convenience of the insured, the insured's family, or the provider.

99. A patient has two health insurance policies: Medicare and a Medicare supplement. Which of the following statements is true?

    a. The patient receives any monies paid by the insurance companies over and above the charges.

    b. Coordination of benefits is necessary to determine which policy is primary and which is secondary so that there is no duplication of payments.

    c. The decision on which company is primary is based on remittance advice.

    d. The patient should not have a Medicare supplement.

100. What system reimburses hospitals a predetermined amount for each Medicare inpatient admission?

    a. APR-DRG

    b. DRG

    c. APC

    d. RUG

101. Medicare defines fraud as _____.

    a. Billing practices that are inconsistent with generally acceptable fiscal policies

    b. Making unintentional billing errors

    c. Accurately representing the types of services provided, dates of services, or identity of the patient

    d. Intentional deception or misrepresentation that results in an unauthorized benefit to an individual

102. Which governmental agency develops an annual work plan that delineates the specific target areas for Medicare that will be monitored in a given year?

    a. Centers for Medicare and Medicaid (CMS)

    b. Federal Bureau of Investigation (FBI)

    c. Office of Inspector General (OIG)

    d. Defense Criminal Investigative Service (DCIS)

103. What is one way that physicians can prevent or minimize potentially abusive or fraudulent activities?

    a. Developing a compliance plan

    b. Upcoding

    c. Unbundling

    d. Billing for noncovered services

104. The MS-DRG system creates a hospital's case-mix index (types or categories of patients treated by the hospital) based on the relative weights of the MS-DRG. The case mix can be figured by multiplying the relative weight of each MS-DRG by the number of _____ within that MS-DRG.

    a. Admissions

    b. Discharges

    c. CCs

    d. MCCs

105. Medicare beneficiaries who have low incomes and limited financial resources may also receive assistance from which federal matching program?

    a. Social Security

    b. Medicare Advantage

    c. Tricare

    d. Medicaid

106. Under the OPPS, on which code set is the APC system primarily based for outpatient procedures and services including devices, drugs, and other covered items?

    a. CPT/HCPCS

    b. ICD-10-CM

    c. CDT

    d. MS-DRG

107. Sometimes hospital departments must work together to solve claims issue errors to prevent them from happening over and over again. What departments would need to work together if an audit found that the claim did not contain the procedure code or charge for a pacemaker insertion?

    a. Health Information and Business Office

    b. Health Information and Materials Management

    c. Health Information, Business Office, and Cardiac Department

    d. Health Information and Radiology

108. Medicare's newest claims processing payment contract entities are referred to as _____.

    a. Recovery audit contractors (RACs)

    b. Medicare administrative contractors (MACs)

    c. Fiscal intermediaries (FIs)

    d. Office of Inspector General contractors (OIGCs)

109. Which of the following best describes the type of coding utilized when a CPT/HCPCS code is assigned directly through the charge description master for claim submission and bypasses the record review and code assignment by the facility coding staff?

    a. Hard coding

    b. Soft coding

    c. Encoder coding

    d. Natural-language processing coding

110. What is a guarantor?

    a. The patient who is an inpatient

    b. The person responsible for the bill, such as a parent

    c. The person who bills the patient, such as the Medicare biller

    d. The patient who is an outpatient

Domain 3   *Health Records and Data Content*

111. Which of the following elements is *not* a component of most patient records?

    a. Patient identification

    b. Clinical history

    c. Financial information

    d. Test results

112. Identify where the following information would be found in the acute-care record: Following induction of an adequate general anesthesia, and with the patient supine on the padded table, the left upper extremity was prepped and draped in the standard fashion.

    a. Anesthesia report

    b. Physician progress notes

    c. Operative report

    d. Recovery room record

113. Identify where the following information would be found in the acute-care record: "CBC: WBC 12.0, RBC 4.65, HGB 14.8, HCT 43.3, MCV 93."

    a. Medical laboratory report

    b. Pathology report

    c. Physical examination

    d. Physician orders

114. Identify where the following information would be found in the acute-care record: "PA and Lateral Chest: The lungs are clear. The heart and mediastinum are normal in size and configuration. There are minor degenerative changes of the lower thoracic spine."

    a. Medical laboratory report

    b. Physical examination

    c. Physician progress note

    d. Radiography report

115. The _____ provided the impetus for standardizing health care records with minimum standards early in the twentieth century:

    a. JCAHO

    b. AHA

    c. ACS

    d. CMS

116. The following is documented in an acute-care record: "Microscopic: Sections are of squamous mucosa with no atypia." Where would this documentation be found?

    a. History

    b. Pathology report

    c. Physical examination

    d. Operation report

117. The following is documented in an acute-care record: "Admit to 3C. Diet: NPO. Meds: Compazine 10 mg IV Q 6 PRN." Where would this documentation be found?

    a. Admission order

    b. History

    c. Physical examination

    d. Progress notes

118. The following is documented in an acute-care record: "38 weeks gestation, Apgars 8/9, 6# 9.8 oz, good cry." Where would this documentation be found?

    a. Admission note

    b. Clinical laboratory

    c. Newborn record

    d. Physician order

119. The following is documented in an acute-care record: "Atrial fibrillation with rapid ventricular response, left axis deviation, left bundle branch block." Where would this documentation be found?

    a. Admission order

    b. Clinical laboratory report

    c. ECG report

    d. Radiology report

120. The regulations for health care record content and documentation, guidelines and regulations for which facilities are allowed to take part in or join the Medicare and Medicaid programs is:

    a. Medical Staff Bylaws

    b. Conditions of Participation

    c. Joint Commission Rules

    d. American College of Surgeon's Regulations

121. The following is documented in an acute-care record: "Spoke to the attending re: my assessment. Provided adoption and counseling information. Spoke to CPS re: referral. Case manager to meet with patient and family." Where would this documentation be found?

    a. Admission note

    b. Nursing note

    c. Physician progress note

    d. Social work note

122. Mary Smith, RHIA, has been charged with the responsibility of designing a data collection form to be used on admission of a patient to the acute-care hospital in which she works. The first resource that she should use is _____.

    a. UHDDS

    b. UACDS

    c. MDS

    d. ORYX

123. Even though state laws may be more stringent, CMS requires acute healthcare records to be maintained by the acute health care organization for:

    a. Ten years

    b. At least 5 years

    c. Minimum of 25 years

    d. Permanent access

124. A notation for a diabetic patient in a physician progress note reads: "Occasionally gets hungry. No insulin reactions. Says she is following her diabetic diet." Which part of a POMR progress note would this notation be written?

    a. Subjective

    b. Objective

    c. Assessment

    d. Plan

125. A notation for a diabetic patient in a physician progress note reads: "FBS 110 mg%, urine sugar, no acetone." Which part of a POMR progress note would this notation be written?

    a. Subjective

    b. Objective

    c. Assessment

    d. Plan

126. A notation for a hypertensive patient in a physician ambulatory care progress note reads: "Continue with Diuril, 500 mgs once daily. Return visit in 2 weeks." Which part of a POMR progress note would this notation be written?

    a. Subjective

    b. Objective

    c. Assessment

    d. Plan

127. A notation for a hypertensive patient in a physician ambulatory care progress note reads: "Blood pressure adequately controlled." Which part of a POMR progress note would this notation be written?

    a. Subjective

    b. Objective

    c. Assessment

    d. Plan

128. Reviewing the health record for missing signatures, missing medical reports, and ensuring that all documents belong in the health record is an example of _____ review.

    a. Quantitative

    b. Qualitative

    c. Statistical

    d. Outcomes

129. Dr. Jones entered a progress note in a patient's health record 24 hours after he visited the patient. Which quality element is missing from the progress note?

    a. Data completeness

    b. Data relevancy

    c. Data currency

    d. Data precision

130. The admitting data of Mrs. Smith's health record indicated that her birth date was March 21, 1948. On the discharge summary, Mrs. Smith's birth date was recorded as July 21, 1948. Which quality element is missing from Mrs. Smith's health record?

    a. Data completeness

    b. Data consistency

    c. Data accessibility

    d. Data comprehensiveness

131. Which of the following is an example of clinical data?

    a. Admitting diagnosis

    b. Date and time of admission

    c. Insurance information

    d. Health record number

132. Documentation of aides who assist a patient with activities of daily living, bathing, laundry, and cleaning would be found in which type of specialty record?

    a. Home health

    b. Behavioral health

    c. End-stage renal disease

    d. Rehabilitative care

133. Which of the following materials is *not* documented in an emergency care record?

    a. Patient's instructions at discharge

    b. Time and means of the patient's arrival

    c. Patient's complete medical history

    d. Emergency care administered before arrival at the facility

134. Which of the following provides macroscopic and microscopic information about tissue removed during an operative procedure?

    a. Anesthesia report

    b. Laboratory report

    c. Operative report

    d. Pathology report

135. What is the defining characteristic of an integrated health record format?

    a. Each section of the record is maintained by the patient care department that provided the care.

    b. Integrated health records are intended to be used in ambulatory settings.

    c. Integrated health records include both paper forms and computer printouts.

    d. Integrated health record components are arranged in strict chronological order.

136. Which of the following represents documentation of the patient's current and past health status?

    a. Physical examination

    b. Medical history

    c. Physician orders

    d. Patient consent

137. Which of the following contains the physician's findings based on an examination of the patient?

    a. Physical examination

    b. Discharge summary

    c. Medical history

    d. Patient instructions

138. What is the function of a consultation report?

    a. Provides a chronological summary of the patient's medical history and illness

    b. Documents opinions about the patient's condition from the perspective of a physician not previously involved in the patient's care

    c. Concisely summarizes the patient's treatment and stay in the hospital

    d. Documents the physician's instructions to other parties involved in providing care to a patient

139. What is the function of physician's orders?

    a. Provide a chronological summary of the patient's illness and treatment

    b. Document the patient's current and past health status

    c. Document the physician's instructions to other parties involved in providing care to a patient

    d. Document the provider's follow-up care instructions given to the patient or patient's caregiver

140. In the acute care facility, the patient identity management tool that ensures that the right patient connects to the right information relies on:

    a. Master Patient Index (MPI)

    b. Case Mix Index (CMI)

    c. The Organization's clinical staff

    d. Cancer Registry

Domain 4 *Compliance*

141. In a joint effort of the Department of Health and Human Services (DHHS), Office of Inspector General (OIG), Centers for Medicare and Medicaid Services (CMS), and Administration on Aging (AOA), which program was released in 1995 to target fraud and abuse among healthcare providers?

    a. Operation Restore Trust

    b. Medicare Integrity Program

    c. Tax Equity and Fiscal Responsibility Act (TEFRA)

    d. Medicare and Medicaid Patient and Program Protection Act

142. All of the following should be part of the core areas of a coding compliance plan *except*:

    a. Physician query process

    b. Correct use of encoder software

    c. Coding diagnoses supported by medical record documentation

    d. Tracking length of stay

143. Common forms of fraud and abuse include all of the following *except*:

    a. Upcoding

    b. Unbundling or "exploding" charges

    c. Refiling claims after denials

    d. Billing for services not furnished to patients

144. What is the primary use of the case-mix index?

    a. Benchmark of emergency room levels

    b. Defines how a hospital compares to peers and whether the facility is at risk

    c. Audit of APCS and the comparison to same-size hospitals

    d. A tool for the coding manager to compare coder productivity

145. A(n) _____ is considered the most innocent of improper payments because there is no intent to falsely receive a payment from the payer:

    a. Fraud

    b. Abuse

    c. Mistake

    d. Error claim

146. To combat fraud and abuse in coding, one strategy is to:

    a. Use computer assisted coding (CAC)

    b. Unbundle codes

    c. Use best practices to write a query to clarify documentation

    d. Ensure the meaningful use incentive program

147. What is the process used to transform text into an unintelligible string of characters that can be transmitted via communications media with a high degree of security and then decrypted when it reaches a secure destination?

    a. Distortion

    b. Extrication

    c. Encryption

    d. Encoded

148. Using uniform terminology is a way to improve:

    a. Validity

    b. Data timeliness

    c. Audit trails

    d. Data reliability

149. The _____ mandated the development of standards for electronic medical records.

    a. Medicare and Medicaid legislation of 1965

    b. Prospective Payment Act of 1983

    c. Health Insurance Portability and Accountability Act (HIPAA) of 1996

    d. Balanced Budget Act of 1997

150. Messaging standards for electronic data interchange in healthcare have been developed by:

    a. HL7

    b. IEE

    c. The Joint Commission

    d. CMS

151. What is the incentive to improve the quality of clinical outcomes using the electronic health record that could result in additional reimbursement or eligibility for grants or other subsidies to support further HIT efforts?

    a. Pay for performance and quality

    b. Patient referrals

    c. Payer of last resort

    d. Performance evaluations

152. A threat to data security is _____.

    a. Encryption

    b. Malware

    c. Audit trail

    d. Data quality

153. Data security refers to _____.

    a. Guaranteeing privacy

    b. Controlling access

    c. Using uniform terminology

    d. Transparency

154. A record of all transactions in the computer system that is maintained and reviewed for unauthorized access is called a(n) _____.

    a. Security breach

    b. Audit trail

    c. Unauthorized access

    d. Privacy trail

155. The _____ permits penalties to be awarded to those who intentionally submit fraudulent claims to the US government:

    a. Anti-kickback statute

    b. Balanced budget act of 1997

    c. False Claims Act

    d. HIPAA

156. Performance counseling usually begins with which of the following?

    a. Submitting an action plan of steps the employee will do to resolve the issue and improve performance

    b. Job termination

    c. Informal counseling or verbal warning

    d. Put the coder on unpaid leave of absence

157. A health information technician (HIT) is hired as the chief compliance officer for a large group practice. In evaluating the current program, the HIT learns that there are written standards of conduct and policies and procedures that address specific areas of potential fraud as well as audits in place to monitor compliance. Which of the following should the compliance officer also ensure are in place?

    a. Compliance program education and training programs for all employees in the organization

    b. Establishment of a hotline to receive complaints and adoption of procedures to protect whistleblowers from retaliation

    c. Adopt procedures to adequately identify individuals who make complaints so that appropriate follow-up can be conducted

    d. Establish a corporate compliance committee who report directly to the CFO

158. In developing a coding compliance program, which of the following would not be ordinarily included as participants in coding compliance education?

    a. Current coding personnel

    b. Medical staff

    c. Newly hired coding personnel

    d. Nursing staff

159. Which of the following issues compliance program guidance?

    a. AHIMA

    b. CMS

    c. Federal Register

    d. HHS Office of Inspector General (OIG)

160. The practice of assigning a diagnosis or procedure code specifically for the purpose of obtaining a higher level of payment is called _____.

    a. Billing

    b. Unbundling

    c. Upcoding

    d. Unnecessary service

161. This person designs, implements, and maintains a program that ensures conformity to all types of regulatory and voluntary accreditation requirements governing the provision of healthcare products or services _____.

    a. General Counsel

    b. Health Information Director

    c. Privacy Officer

    d. Compliance Officer

162. The HIM department is planning to scan medical record documentation. The project includes the scanning of documentation such as history and physicals, physician orders, operative reports, and nursing notes. Which of the following methods of scanning would be best to help HIM professionals monitor the completeness of health records during a patient's hospitalization?

    a. Ad hoc

    b. Concurrent

    c. Retrospective

    d. Post discharge

163. Which of the following laws created the Healthcare Integrity and Protection Data Bank?

    a. Health Information Portability and Accountability Act

    b. American Recovery and Reinvestment Act

    c. Consolidate Omnibus Budget Reconciliation Act

    d. Healthcare Quality Improvement Act

164. The Office of Inspector General's (OIG's) strategic plan includes four goals:

    a. Reduce risk, prevent criminal conduct, enforce laws and maintain ethics in health care.

    b. Fight fraud, waste and abuse; promise quality and safety, secure and advance future innovations in healthcare.

    c. Prevent criminal conduct; promulgate quality and safety; educate medical staff; and oversee disciplinary actions.

    d. Promote quality and safety, education for patients and clinical staff and advance pharmaceuticals' best use.

165. In 2009, the HHS and DOJ created the _____ to prevent waste, fraud and abuse, reduce health care costs and improve the quality of care provided to Medicare patient:

    a. Office of Inspector General (OIG)

    b. Recovery Audit Contractor (RAC)

    c. Quality Improvement Organization and Enforcement (QIO)

    d. Health Care Fraud Prevention Team (HEAT)

166. An accounting of disclosures must include disclosures _____.

    a. For use in law enforcement requests

    b. To any patient family member who makes a request

    c. To any individual who requested the information

    d. Made for public health reporting purposes

167. Notices of privacy practices must be available at the site where the individual is treated and:

    a. Must be posted next to the entrance

    b. Must be posted in a prominent place where it is reasonable to expect that patients will read them

    c. May be posted anywhere at the site

    d. Do not have to be posted at the site

168. Calling out patient names in a physician's office is:

    a. An incidental disclosure

    b. Not subject to the "minimum necessary" requirement

    c. A disclosure for payment purposes

    d. A HIPAA violation

Domain 5 | *Information Technologies*

169. Which of the following is *not* an element of data quality?

    a. Accessibility

    b. Data backup

    c. Precision

    d. Relevancy

170. The protection measures and tools for safeguarding information and information systems is a definition of _____.

    a. Confidentiality

    b. Data security

    c. Informational privacy

    d. Informational access control

171. Computer software programs that assist in the assignment of codes used with diagnostic and procedural classifications are called _____.

    a. Natural-language processing systems

    b. Monitoring/audit programs

    c. Encoders

    d. Concept, description, and relationship tables

172. A special webpage that offers secure access to data is called a(n) _____.

    a. Access control

    b. Home page

    c. Intranet

    d. Portal

173. One form of _____ uses software to aid the physician in selecting the correct code with processes such as drop-down boxes or the use of touch-screen terminals.

    a. Integrated workflow processes

    b. Computer-assisted coding

    c. Electronic document management system

    d. Speech recognition system

174. One form of _____ computer-assisted coding may use, which means that digital text from online documents stored in the information system is read directly by the software, which then suggests codes to match the documentation.

    a. Encoded vocabulary

    b. Natural-language processing

    c. Data exchange standards

    d. Structured reports

175. The _____ was issued by the Office of the National Coordinator (ONC) for health information technology to be a resource to the nation as a vision and reference:

    a. Health Information Technology for Economic and Clinical Health (HITECH)

    b. American Recovery and Reinvestment Act (ARRA)

    c. Meaningful Use (MU) Program

    d. Federal Health Information Technology Strategic Plan 2015–2020

176. Electronic systems used by nurses and physicians to document assessments and findings are called:

    a. Computerized provider order entry

    b. Electronic document management systems

    c. Electronic medication administration records

    d. Electronic patient care charting

177. Data definition refers to:

    a. Meaning of data

    b. Completeness of data

    c. Consistency of data

    d. Detail of data

178. An encoder that is built using expert system techniques such as rule-based systems is a(n):

    a. Encoder interface

    b. Logic-based encoder

    c. Automated code book encoder

    d. Grouper

179. Good encoding software should include _____ to ensure data quality.

    a. Edit checks

    b. Voice recognition

    c. Reimbursement technology

    d. Passwords

180. The communication and network technologies connections, known as _____, are used by providers to submit orders for medications and lab tests.

    a. Computerized order entry system (CPOE)

    b. Bar code medication administration record (BC-MAR)

    c. Electronic Health Record (EHR)

    d. Personal health record (PHR)

181. Which of the following make data entry easier but may harm data quality?

    a. Use of templates

    b. Copy and paste

    c. Drop-down boxes

    d. Structured data

182. A transition technology used by many hospitals to increase access to medical record content is _____.

    a. EHR (electronic health record)

    b. EDMS (electronic document management system)

    c. ESA (electronic signature authentication)

    d. PACS (picture archiving and communication system)

183. This system will require the author to sign onto the system using a user ID and password to complete the entries made.

    a. Digital dictation

    b. Electronic signature authentication

    c. Single sign on technology

    d. Clinical data repository

184. Coders will assign codes that have been selected into a computer program called a(n) _____ to assign the patient's case to the correct group based on ICD-10-CM/PCS and/or CPT/HCPCS codes.

    a. Encoder

    b. Computer-assisted coding

    c. Natural-language processor

    d. Grouper

Domain 6 *Confidentiality and Privacy*

185. What is the legal term used to define the protection of health information in a patient–provider relationship?

    a. Access

    b. Confidentiality

    c. Privacy

    d. Security

186. The Uniform Health Care Decisions Act ranks the next-of-kin in the following order for medical decision-making purposes _____.

    a. Adult sibling; adult child; spouse; parent

    b. Parent; spouse; adult child; adult sibling

    c. Spouse; parent; adult sibling; adult child

    d. Spouse; adult child; parent; adult sibling

187. Which of the following is a direct command that requires an individual or a representative of an organization to appear in court or to present an object to the court?

    a. Judicial decision

    b. Subpoena

    c. Credential

    d. Regulation

188. Exceptions to the consent requirement include _____.

    a. Medical emergencies

    b. Provider discretion

    c. Implied consent

    d. Informed consent

189. The term *minimum necessary* means that healthcare providers and other covered entities must limit use, access, and disclosure to the minimum necessary to _____.

    a. Satisfy one's curiosity

    b. Accomplish the intended purpose

    c. Treat an individual

    d. Perform research

190. A well-informed patient will know that the HIPAA Privacy Rule requires that individuals be able to _____.

    a. Request restrictions on certain uses and disclosures of PHI

    b. Remove their record from the facility

    c. Deny provider changes to their PHI

    d. Delete portions of the record they think are incorrect

191. Written or spoken permission to proceed with care is classified as _____.

    a. An advanced directive

    b. Formal consent

    c. Expressed consent

    d. Implied consent

192. The number that has been proposed for use as a unique patient identification number but is controversial because of confidentiality and privacy concerns is the _____.

    a. Social security number

    b. Unique physician identification number

    c. Health record number

    d. National provider identifier

193. Deidentified information _____.

    a. Does identify an individual

    b. Is information from which personal characteristics have been stripped

    c. Can be later constituted or combined to re-identify an individual

    d. Pertains to a person that is identified within the information

194. Which of the following is *not* true of notices of privacy practices?

    a. They must be made available at the site where the individual is treated.

    b. They must be posted in a prominent place.

    c. They must contain content that may not be changed.

    d. They must be prominently posted on the covered entity's website when the entity has one.

195. The Federal Rules of Civil Procedure (FRCP) incorporated the pre-trial process through the creation of:

    a. Bench warrants

    b. Court orders

    c. Depositions

    d. E-discovery

196. Which document directs an individual to bring originals or copies of records to court?

    a. Summons

    b. Subpoena

    c. Subpoena duces tecum

    d. Deposition

197. To comply with HIPAA, under usual circumstances, a covered entity must act on a patient's request to review or copy his or her health information within _____ days.

    a. 10

    b. 20

    c. 30

    d. 60

198. The HIPAA Privacy Rule requires that covered entities must limit use, access, and disclosure of PHI to only the amount needed to accomplish the intended purpose. What concept is this an example of?

    a. Minimum Necessary

    b. Notice of Privacy Practices

    c. Authorization

    d. Consent

199. Which of the following statements is *false*?

    a. A notice of privacy practices must be written in plain language.

    b. Consent for use and disclosure of information must be obtained from every patient.

    c. An authorization does not have to be obtained for uses and disclosures for treatment, payment, and operations.

    d. A notice of privacy practices must give an example of a use or disclosure for healthcare operations.

200. Which of the following statements is *not* true about a business associate agreement?

    a. It prohibits the business associate from using or disclosing PHI for any purpose other than that described in the contract with the covered entity.

    b. It allows the business associate to maintain PHI indefinitely.

    c. It prohibits the business associate from using or disclosing PHI in any way that would violate the HIPAA Privacy Rule.

    d. It requires the business associate to make available all of its books and records relating to PHI use and disclosure to the Department of Health and Human Services or its agents.

EXAM 1

Domain 1 | *Clinical Classification Systems*

1. Identify the ICD-10-CM code for a patient with a subsequent encounter for routine healing of a closed traumatic capital epiphyseal fracture of the left femur.

   a. S79.012A

   b. S79.019D

   c. M84.452D

   d. S79.012D

2. Identify the ICD-10-CM code(s) for neonatal tooth eruption.

   a. K01.1

   b. K00.6, K08.0

   c. K01.0

   d. K00.6

3. Identify CPT code(s) for the following patient. A 35-year-old female undergoes an excision of a 3.0-cm tumor in her forehead. An incision is made through the skin and subcutaneous tissue. The tumor is dissected free of surrounding structures. The wound is closed with interrupted sutures.

   a. 21012

   b. 21012, 12052

   c. 21014

   d. 21014, 12052

4. Identify CPT code(s) for the following Medicare patient. A 67-year-old female undergoes an excision of a breast lesion identified by preoperative placement of radiological marker.

   a. 19101

   b. 19101, 19125

   c. 19125

   d. 19125, 19126

5. Identify the information classified in the fourth digit for the code G30.0.

   a. Alzheimer's disease with early onset

   b. Alzheimer's disease with late onset

   c. Other Alzheimer's disease

   d. Alzheimer's disease, unspecified

6. Identify the ICD-10-PCS code(s) for insertion of dual chamber cardiac pacemaker battery via an incision in the subcutaneous tissue of the chest wall, and percutaneous transvenous insertion of right atrial and right ventricular leads.

   a. 0JH606Z, 02H73JZ, 02HL3JZ

   b. 0WH80YZ, 02H63JZ, 02HK3JZ

   c. 0WH80YZ, 02H73JZ, 02HL3JZ

   d. 0JH606Z, 02H63JZ, 02HK3JZ

7. Identify the correct ICD-10-PCS code(s) for replacement of an old dual pacemaker with a new dual pacemaker in the subcutaneous tissue of the chest wall via incisional approach.

   a. 0JPT0PZ, 0JH606Z

   b. 0JH606Z

   c. 0JWT0PZ

   d. 0JPT3PZ, 0JH634Z

8. Identify the appropriate ICD-10-CM code(s) for Mobitz type I and II heart block.

   a. I44.7, I45.19

   b. I44.1

   c. I45.0, I45.2

   d. I45.10

9. Identify the appropriate ICD-10-CM and ICD-10-PCS code(s) for cardiac pacemaker pulse generator check.

   a. Z45.010, 4B02XSZ

   b. Z45.018, 4B02XTZ

   c. T82.121A, 4B02XSZ

   d. Z45.010, 4B02XTZ

10. When both hypertension and a condition classifiable to category N18, Chronic kidney disease (CKD), are present, assign codes from category:

    a. I13, Hypertensive heart and chronic kidney disease

    b. I15, Secondary Hypertension

    c. I12, Hypertensive chronic kidney disease

    d. I27.0, Primary Pulmonary Hypertension

11. Identify the appropriate ICD-10-PCS code(s) for a coronary artery bypass of two sites, one using the left internal mammary artery to the left proximal anterior descending artery, and one using the right internal mammary artery to the distal left anterior descending artery, both done via thoracotomy.

    a. 02104K8, 02104K9

    b. 02110A8, 02110A9

    c. 02100Z8, 02100Z9

    d. 021109W

12. Coronary arteriography serves as a diagnostic tool in detecting obstruction within the coronary arteries. Identify the technique using two catheters inserted percutaneously through the femoral artery.

    a. Brachial

    b. Stones

    c. Judkins

    d. Femoral

13. Identify the correct ICD-10-CM code(s) for a patient who arrives at the hospital for outpatient laboratory services ordered by the physician to monitor the patient's Coumadin levels. A prothrombin time (PT) is performed to check the patient's long-term use of his anticoagulant treatment.

    a. Z51.81, Z79.01

    b. Z51.81, Z79.02

    c. Z79.01, R79.1

    d. Z79.01

14. Identify the CPT code(s) for the following patient: A 47-year-old male presented to the hospital for a complete wrist fusion which is done using a graft from the iliac crest.

    a. 25800

    b. 25810

    c. 25825, 20900

    d. 25830

15. Identify the CPT code(s) for the following patient: A 2-year-old boy presented to the hospital to have his gastrostomy tube changed repositioned under fluoroscopic guidance.

    a. 43752

    b. 43761

    c. 43761, 76000

    d. 49450

16. Identify the term ICD-10-CM uses for the following definition: "the expulsion of some, but not all, of the products of conception from the uterus."

    a. Spontaneous abortion

    b. Therapeutic abortion

    c. Incomplete abortion

    d. Complete abortion

17. Identify the ICD-10-CM code(s) for the following: threatened abortion with hemorrhage at 15 weeks; home undelivered.

    a. O20.0, O20.9

    b. O20.0, Z3A.15

    c. O20.8

    d. O20.8, Z3A.15

18. Identify the ICD-10-CM and ICD-10-PCS code(s) for the following: 40 week gestation, term pregnancy with poor cervical dilatation; low uterine cesarean delivery, open approach, with single liveborn female.

    a. O62.0, Z3A.40, Z37.0, 10D00Z1

    b. O62.2, 101D00Z0

    c. O62.0, Z3A.40, 10D00Z0

    d. O62.2, Z37.0, 10D00Z1

19. Identify the ICD-10-CM code for diaper rash in elderly patient.

    a. L21.9

    b. L22

    c. R21

    d. L74.3

20. For ulcers that were present on admission but healed at the time of discharge, assign the code for the site and stage of the pressure ulcer _____.

    a. According to the discharge condition

    b. According to the nursing progress notes

    c. According to the condition at time of admission

    d. As documented in the Discharge Summary

21. Identify the ICD-10-CM code(s) for primary localized osteoarthritis of bilateral hips.

    a. M16.11, M16.12

    b. M16.0

    c. M16.4

    d. M16.2

22. Identify the ICD-10-CM code for chondromalacia of the left patella.

    a. M22.42

    b. M22.8X2

    c. M22.92

    d. M94.262

23. Identify the ICD-10-CM code(s) for acute osteomyelitis of the right index finger due to *Staphylococcus aureus*.

    a. M86.14

    b. M86.149, B95.61

    c. M86.141, A49.01

    d. M86.141, B95.61

24. Identify the ICD-10-CM code(s) for a liveborn male infant, transferred to another hospital for care of tetralogy of Fallot:

    a. Q21.3

    b. Z38.01, Q21.0

    c. Q21.0, Z38.00

    d. Z38.00, Q21.3

25. Identify the ICD-10-CM code(s) for other specified aplastic anemia secondary to adverse effect of chemotherapy, initial encounter.

    a. D61.1

    b. D61.1, T45.1X5A

    c. D64.9

    d. D63.0

26. Identify the ICD-10-CM code(s) for the following: A 6-month-old child is scheduled for a clinic visit for a routine well-child examination. The physician documents, "well child, born premature."

    a. Z00.00, P07.30

    b. Z00.129

    c. Z00.129, P07.30

    d. Z00.129, O60.10X0

27. Identify the ICD-10-CM code for ventricular diastolic dysfunction.

    a. I50.1

    b. I50.30

    c. I50.9

    d. I51.9

28. Identify the chapter in which certain signs and symptoms of breast disease, such as mastodynia, induration of breast, and nipple discharge, are included.

    a. Chapter 2 Neoplasms

    b. Chapter 12 Diseases of the skin and subcutaneous tissue

    c. Chapter 14 Diseases of the genitourinary system

    d. Chapter 18 Symptoms, signs and abnormal clinical and laboratory findings, not elsewhere classified

29. Which of the following is the correct ICD-10-PCS code for a Mayo operation known as a bunionectomy? An incision was made in the right foot and a portion of the first metatarsal head was removed.

    a. 0SRP0JZ

    b. 0STP0ZZ

    c. 0QBN0ZZ

    d. 0QTN0ZZ

30. If a patient is admitted with a pressure ulcer at one stage and it progresses to a higher stage, _____.

    a. Assign two separate codes, one code for the site and stage of the ulcer on admission and a second code for the same ulcer site and the highest stage reported during the stay.

    b. Assign only the highest stage documented during the stay.

    c. Assign only the stage of the ulcer on admission.

    d. Query the attending physician for the appropriate site and stage of the pressure ulcer.

31. Which of the following is (are) the correct ICD-10-PCS code(s) for laparoscopic cholecystectomy? The entire gallbladder was removed.

    a. 0FT40ZZ

    b. 0FT40ZZ, 0FJ44ZZ

    c. 0FT44ZZ, 0FJ44ZZ

    d. 0FT44ZZ

32. Which of the following is (are) the correct ICD-10-PCS code(s) for cystoscopy with diagnostic biopsy of the bladder?

    a. 0TBB7ZX

    b. 0TJB8ZZ, 0TBB8ZX

    c. 0TBB8ZX

    d. 0TBB8ZZ

Domain 2 *Reimbursement Methodologies*

33. Which of the following software applications would be used to aid in the coding function in a physician's office?

    a. Grouper

    b. Encoder

    c. Pricer

    d. Diagnosis calculator

34. Which payment system was introduced in 1992 and replaced Medicare's customary, prevailing, and reasonable (CPR) payment system?

    a. Diagnosis-related groups

    b. Resource-based relative value scale system

    c. Long-term care drugs

    d. Resource utilization groups

35. The health care program for active duty members of the military and other qualified family members is:

    a. Children's Health Insurance Program (CHIP)

    b. V.A. Funding Inc.

    c. Tricare

    d. Worker's Compensation

36. What is the best reference tool to determine how CPT codes should be assigned?

    a. Local coverage determination from Medicare

    b. American Medical Association's *CPT Assistant* newsletter

    c. American Hospital Association's *Coding Clinic*

    d. CMS website

37. An electrolyte panel (80051) in the laboratory section of CPT consists of tests for carbon dioxide (82374), chloride (82435), potassium (84132), and sodium (84295). If each of the component codes are reported and billed individually on a claim form, this would be a form of:

    a. Optimizing

    b. Unbundling

    c. Sequencing

    d. Classifying

38. In the laboratory section of CPT, if a group of tests overlaps two or more panels, report the panel that incorporates the greatest number of tests to fulfill the code definition. What would a coder do with the remaining test codes that are not part of a panel?

    a. Report the remaining tests using individual test codes, according to CPT.

    b. Do not report the remaining individual test codes.

    c. Report only those test codes that are part of a panel.

    d. Do not report a test code more than once regardless whether the test was performed twice.

39. The Office of Inspector General (OIG) has identified risk areas for physician practices. One type of risk is "clustering." Identify its definition.

    a. Coding or charging one or two middle levels of service codes exclusively

    b. Billing for a more expensive service than the one actually performed

    c. Billing for noncovered services as if they are covered

    d. Assigning additional codes inherent to the main code

40. The front end of the revenue cycle process does not include:

    a. Enterprise wide scheduling system

    b. Claims appeals

    c. Order tracking system

    d. Financial function system

41. What is the best reference tool for ICD-10-CM/PCS coding advice?

    a. CMS Inpatient Prospective Payment System (IPPS)

    b. CMS ICD-10-CM and ICD-10-PCS Coding Guidelines

    c. AHA's *Coding Clinic for ICD-10-CM/PCS*

    d. National Correct Coding Initiative (NCCI)

42. CMS developed medically unlikely edits (MUEs) to prevent providers from billing units of services greater than the norm would indicate. These MUEs were implemented on January 1, 2007, and are applied to which code set?

    a. Diagnosis-related groups

    b. HCPCS/CPT codes

    c. ICD-10-CM/PCS diagnosis and procedure codes

    d. Resource utilization groups

43. Several key principles require appropriate physician documentation to secure payment from the insurer. Which answer (listed here) fails to impact payment based on physician responsibility?

    a. The health record should be complete and legible.

    b. The rationale for ordering diagnostic and other ancillary services should be documented or easily inferred.

    c. Documenting the charges and services on the itemized bill.

    d. The patient's progress and response to treatment and any revision in the treatment plan and diagnoses should be documented.

44. The documentation of each patient encounter should include the following to secure payment from the insurer *except* _____.

    a. The reason for the encounter and the patient's relevant history, physical examination, and prior diagnostic test results

    b. A patient assessment, clinical impression, or diagnosis

    c. A plan of care

    d. The identity of the patient's nearest relative and emergency contact number

45. Two patients were hospitalized with bacterial pneumonia. One patient was hospitalized for three days, and the other patient was hospitalized for 30 days. Both cases result in the same DRG with different lengths of stay. Which answer most closely describes how the hospital will be reimbursed?

    a. The hospital will receive the same DRG for both patients but additional reimbursement will be allowed for the patient who stayed 30 days because the length of stay was greater than the geometric length of stay for this DRG.

    b. The hospital will receive the same reimbursement for the same DRG regardless of the length of stay.

    c. The hospital can appeal the payment for the patient who was in the hospital for 30 days because the cost of care was significantly higher than the average length of stay for the DRG payment.

    d. The hospital will receive a day outlier for the patient who was hospitalized for 30 days.

46. Which one of the following statements is true?

    a. The higher the relative weight, the higher the payment rates.

    b. The lower the relative weight, the higher the payment rates.

    c. The lower the relative weight, the sicker the patient.

    d. The higher the relative weight, the lesser reimbursement due the facility.

47. Which classification system is in place to reimburse home health agencies?

    a. MS-DRGs

    b. RUGs

    c. HHRGs

    d. APCs

48. What reimbursement system uses the Medicare fee schedule?

    a. APCs

    b. MS-DRGs

    c. RBRVS

    d. RUG-III

49. MS diagnostic-related groups are organized into:

    a. Case-mix classifications

    b. Geographic practice cost indices

    c. Major diagnostic categories

    d. Resource-based relative values

50. Which of the following hospitals are excluded from the Medicare acute-care prospective payment system?

    a. Children's

    b. Small community

    c. Tertiary

    d. Trauma

51. CMS identified conditions that are not present on admission and could be "reasonably preventable." Hospitals are not allowed to receive additional payment for these conditions when the condition is present on admission. What are these conditions called?

    a. Conditions of Participation

    b. Present on admission

    c. Hospital-acquired conditions

    d. Hospital-acquired infection

52. Which of the following fails to meet the CMS classification of a hospital-acquired condition?

    a. Foreign object retained after surgery

    b. Air embolism

    c. Gram-negative pneumonia

    d. Blood incompatibility

53. Which of the following fails to meet the CMS classification of a hospital-acquired condition?

    a. Stage I pressure ulcers

    b. Falls and trauma

    c. Catheter-associated infection

    d. Vascular catheter–associated infection

54. The electronic claim format (837I) replaces which paper billing form?

    a. CMS-1500

    b. CMS-1450 (UB-04)

    c. UB-92

    d. CMS-1400

55. This is a statement sent by third-party payers to the patient to explain services provided, amounts billed, and payments made by the health plan.

    a. Coordination of benefits (COB)

    b. Explanation of benefits (EOB)

    c. Medicare summary notice (MSN)

    d. Remittance advice (RA)

Domain 3 | *Health Records and Data Content*

56. An outpatient clinic is reviewing the functionality of a computer system it is considering purchasing. Which of the following datasets should the clinic consult to ensure all the federally required data elements for Medicare and Medicaid outpatient clinical encounters are collected by the system?

    a. DEEDS

    b. EMEDS

    c. UACDS

    d. UHDDS

57. Standardizing medical terminology to avoid differences in naming various medical conditions and procedures (such as the synonyms bunionectomy, McBride procedure, and repair of hallus valgus) is one purpose of _____.

    a. Transaction standards

    b. Content and structure standards

    c. Vocabulary standards

    d. Security standards

58. A family practitioner requests the opinion of a physician specialist in endocrinology who reviews the patient's health record and examines the patient. The physician specialist records findings, impressions, and recommendations in which type of report?

    a. Consultation

    b. Medical history

    c. Physical examination

    d. Progress notes

59. Which of the following is *not* a function of the discharge summary?

    a. Providing information about the patient's insurance coverage

    b. Ensuring the continuity of future care

    c. Providing information to support the activities of the medical staff review committee

    d. Providing concise information that can be used to answer information requests

60. Under HIPAA, at the time of admission to the facility or prior to treatment by the provider, patients must be informed about the use of individual identifiable health information by signing the:

    a. Patient Consent Form

    b. Notice of Privacy Practices

    c. Advance Directives

    d. Property and Valuable List

61. A 65-year-old white male was admitted to the hospital on 1/15 complaining of abdominal pain. The attending physician requested an upper GI series and laboratory evaluation of CBC and UA. The x-ray revealed possible cholelithiasis, and the UA showed an increased white blood cell count. The patient was taken to surgery for an exploratory laparoscopy, and a ruptured appendix was discovered. The chief complaint was _____.

    a. Ruptured appendix

    b. Exploratory laparoscopy

    c. Abdominal pain

    d. Cholelithiasis

62. All documentation entered in the medical record relating to the patient's diagnosis and treatment is considered as this type of data:

    a. Clinical

    b. Identification

    c. Secondary

    d. Financial

63. What type of data is exemplified by the insured party's member identification number?

    a. Demographic data

    b. Clinical data

    c. Certification data

    d. Financial data

64. Which part of the problem-oriented medical record is used by many facilities that have not adopted the whole problem-oriented format?

    a. Problem list as an index

    b. Initial plan

    c. SOAP form of progress notes

    d. Database

65. A method of documenting only abnormal or unusual findings or deviations from the prescribed plan of care is _____.

    a. Flow charting

    b. Discharge summary

    c. Charting by exception

    d. Care paths

66. Mildred Smith was admitted from an acute-care hospital to a nursing facility with the following information: "Patient is being admitted for organic brain syndrome." Underneath the diagnosis, her medical information along with her rehabilitation potential was also listed. On which form is this information documented?

    a. Transfer or referral

    b. Release of information

    c. Patient rights acknowledgment

    d. Admitting physical evaluation

67. According to the Joint Commission Accreditation Standards, which document must be placed in the patient's record before a surgical procedure may be performed?

    a. Admission record

    b. Physician's order

    c. Report of history and physical examination

    d. Discharge summary

68. Bob Smith was admitted to Mercy Hospital on June 21. The physical examination was completed on June 23. According to Medicare Conditions of Participation, which statement applies to this situation?

    a. The record is not in compliance because the physical examination must be completed within 24 hours of admission.

    b. The record is not in compliance because the physical examination must be completed within 48 hours of admission.

    c. The record is in compliance because the physical examination must be completed within 48 hours of admission.

    d. The record is in compliance because the physical examination was completed within 72 hours of admission.

69. A health record with deficiencies that is not complete within the timeframe specified in the medical staff rules and regulations is called a(n):

    a. Suspended record

    b. Delinquent record

    c. Pending record

    d. Illegal record

70. The _____ may contain information about diseases among relatives in which heredity may play a role.

    a. Physical examination

    b. History

    c. Laboratory report

    d. Administrative data

Domain 4   *Compliance*

71. To comply with Joint Commission standards, the HIM director wants to ensure that history and physical examinations are documented in the patient's health record no later than 24 hours after admission. Which of the following would be the *best* way to ensure the completeness of health records?

    a. Retrospectively review each patient's medical record to make sure history and physicals are present.

    b. Review each patient's medical record concurrently to make sure history and physicals are present and meet the accreditation standards.

    c. Establish a process to review medical records immediately on discharge.

    d. Do a review of records for all patients discharged in the previous 60 days.

72. Medical record completion compliance is a problem at Community Hospital. The number of incomplete charts often exceeds the standard set by the Joint Commission, risking a type I violation. Previous HIM committee chairpersons tried multiple methods to improve compliance, including suspension of privileges and deactivating the parking garage keycard of any physician in poor standing. To improve compliance, which of the following would be the next step to overcome noncompliance?

    a. Discuss the problem with the hospital CEO, CIO, and CFO.

    b. Call the Joint Commission.

    c. Contact other hospitals to see what methods they use to ensure compliance.

    d. Drop the issue because noncompliance is always a problem.

73. How do accreditation organizations such as the Joint Commission use the health record?

    a. To serve as a source for case study information

    b. To determine whether the documentation supports the provider's claim for reimbursement

    c. To provide healthcare services

    d. To determine whether standards of care are being met

74. Valley High, a skilled nursing facility, wants to become certified to take part in federal government reimbursement programs such as Medicare. What standards must the facility meet in order to become certified for these programs?

    a. Joint Commission Accreditation Standards

    b. Accreditation Association for Ambulatory Healthcare Standards

    c. Conditions of Participation

    d. Outcomes and Assessment Information Set

75. An effective compliance program should include some basic elements to comply with state and federal laws. These include policies, procedures and standards of conduct; the identification of a compliance officer and committee; education of staff; establishment of communication channels; performance of internal monitoring; corrective action when a problem is identified; and _____:

    a. Clinical documentation strategies

    b. Penalties for non-compliance of standards

    c. Improving the accuracy of health claims

    d. External audits

76. This document includes a microscopic description of tissue excised during surgery:

    a. Recovery room record

    b. Pathology report

    c. Operative report

    d. Discharge summary

77. When the physician does not specify the method used to remove a lesion during an endoscopy, what is the appropriate procedure?

    a. Assign the removal by snare technique code.

    b. Assign the removal by hot biopsy forceps code.

    c. Assign the ablation code.

    d. Query the physician as to the method used.

78. The Medicare Modernization Act of 2003 (MMA) launched a Medicare payment and recovery demonstration project that would later develop into recovery audit contractors (RACs) serving as a means to ensure correct payments under Medicare. During the demonstration program, the contractors were able to identify _____ of dollars in improper payments.

    a. Hundreds

    b. Thousands

    c. Millions

    d. Billions

79. Corporate compliance programs were released by the OIG for hospitals to develop and implement their own compliance programs. All of the following *except* _____ are basic elements of a corporate compliance program.

    a. Designation of a chief compliance officer

    b. Implementation of regular and effective education and training programs for all employees

    c. Medical staff appointee for documentation compliance

    d. The use of audits or other evaluation techniques to monitor compliance

80. Which of the following programs has been in place in hospitals for years and has been required by the Medicare and Medicaid programs and accreditation standards?

    a. Internal DRG audits

    b. Peer review

    c. Managed care

    d. Quality improvement

81. Each year the OIG develops a work plan that details areas of compliance it will be investigating for that year. What is the expectation of the hospital in relation to the OIG work plan?

    a. Hospitals are required to follow the same work plan and deploy audits based on that work plan.

    b. Hospitals should plan their compliance and auditing projects around the OIG work plan to ensure they are in compliance with the target areas in the plan.

    c. Hospitals must not develop their audits based on the OIG work plan; rather, they must develop their own and look for high-risk areas that need improvement.

    d. Hospitals must use the plan developed by their state hospital association that is specific to state laws and compliance activities.

82. HIM coding professionals and the organizations that employ them have the responsibility to not tolerate behavior that adversely affects data quality. Which of the following is an example of behavior that should *not* be tolerated?

    a. Omit codes that reflect negatively on quality and patient safety measurement.

    b. Follow-up on and monitor identified problems.

    c. Evaluate and trend diagnoses and procedure code selections.

    d. Report data quality review results to organizational leadership, compliance staff, and the medical staff.

83. The OIG believes that compliance programs have benefits in addition to submitting accurate claims. This includes all of the following *except* _____.

    a. Demonstration of the organization's commitment to responsible conduct toward employees and the community

    b. Provision of a more accurate view of behavior relating to fraud and abuse

    c. Increased potential for criminal and unethical conduct

    d. Improvements in the quality of patient care

84. An individual stole and used another person's insurance information to obtain medical care. This action would be considered _____.

    a. Violation of bioethics

    b. Fraud and abuse

    c. Medical identity theft

    d. Abuse

85. A hospital HIM department wants to purchase an electronic system that records the location of health records removed from the filing system and documents the date of their return to the HIM department. Which of the following electronic systems would fulfill this purpose?

    a. Chart deficiency system

    b. Chart tracking system

    c. Chart abstracting system

    d. Chart encoder

86. What does an audit trail check for?

    a. Unauthorized access to a system

    b. Loss of data

    c. Presence of a virus

    d. Successful completion of a backup

87. An individual designated as an inpatient coder may have access to an electronic medical record to code the record. Under what access security mechanism is the coder allowed access to the system?

    a. Role-based

    b. User-based

    c. Context-based

    d. Situation-based

88. What software will prompt the user through a variety of questions and choices based on the clinical terminology entered to assist the coder in selecting the most appropriate code?

    a. Logic-based encoder

    b. Automated code book

    c. Speech recognition

    d. Natural-language processing

89. The technology commonly used for automated claims processing (sending bills directly to third-party payers) is _____.

    a. Optical character recognition

    b. Bar coding

    c. Neural networks

    d. Electronic data interchange

90. The final state that demonstrates effective adoption for systems operations along with understanding and appropriate use is:

    a. Implementation

    b. Meaningful use

    c. Optimization

    d. Adoption

91. A system that provides alerts and reminders to clinicians is a(n) _____.

    a. Clinical decision support system

    b. Electronic data interchange

    c. Point of care charting system

    d. Knowledge database

92. In what form of health information exchange are data centrally located but physically separated?

    a. Consolidated

    b. Consolidated federated

    c. Centralized

    d. Federated

Domain 6   *Confidentiality and Privacy*

93. A hospital receives a valid request from a patient for copies of his or her medical records. The HIM clerk who is preparing the records removes copies of the patient's records from another hospital where the patient was previously treated. According to HIPAA regulations, was this action correct?

    a. Yes; HIPAA only requires that current records be produced for the patient.

    b. Yes; this is hospital policy over which HIPAA has no control.

    c. No; the records from the previous hospital are considered part of the designated record set and should be given to the patient.

    d. No; the records from the previous hospital are not included in the designated record set but should be released anyway.

94. A patient requests copies of her personal health information on CD. When the patient goes home, she finds that she cannot read the CD on her computer. The patient then requests the hospital to provide the medical records in paper format. How should the hospital respond?

    a. Provide the medical records in paper format

    b. Burn another CD because this is hospital policy

    c. Provide the patient with both paper and CD copies of the medical record

    d. Review the CD copies with the patient on a hospital computer

95. The formal proceeding, where the oral testimony of a party to a lawsuit, including plaintiff, defendant and other relevant witnesses, is known as _____.

    a. Subpoena

    b. Interrogatory

    c. Deposition

    d. Discovery

96. The release of information function requires the HIM professional to have knowledge of
_____.

    a. Clinical coding principles

    b. Database development

    c. Federal and state confidentiality laws

    d. Human resource management

97. The Medical Record Committee is reviewing the privacy policies for a large outpatient clinic. One of the members of the committee remarks that he feels the clinic's practice of calling out a patient's full name in the waiting room is not in compliance with HIPAA regulations and that only the patient's first name should be used. Other committee members disagree with this assessment. What should the HIM director advise the committee?

    a. HIPAA does not allow a patient's name to be announced in a waiting room.

    b. There is no HIPAA violation for announcing a patient's name, but the committee may want to consider implementing practices that might reduce this practice.

    c. HIPAA allows only the use of the patient's first name.

    d. HIPAA requires that patients be given numbers and only the number be announced.

98. The right of an individual to keep information about himself or herself from being disclosed to anyone is a definition of _____.

    a. Confidentiality

    b. Privacy

    c. Integrity

    d. Security

99. The HIM manager is concerned about whether the data transmitted across the hospital network is altered during the transmission. The concept that concerns the HIM manager is _____.

    a. Admissibility

    b. Disclosures

    c. Availability

    d. Data integrity

100. The CIA of security includes confidentiality, data integrity, and data _____.

    a. Accessibility

    b. Authentication

    c. Accuracy

    d. Availability

EXAM 2

Domain 1 *Clinical Classification Systems*

1. Identify the correct ICD-10-CM diagnosis code(s) and sequencing for the following: patient with a scar on the right hand secondary to a laceration sustained two years ago.

   a. L90.5

   b. S61.411S

   c. L90.5, S61.411S

   d. S61.411S, L90.5

2. Identify the correct ICD-10-CM diagnosis code(s) and sequencing for the following: patient with dysphasia secondary to a previous cerebral infarction.

   a. R13.10, I69.391

   b. R47.02, I69.391

   c. I69.391, R13.10

   d. R13.10, I69.398

3. Identify the correct ICD-10-CM diagnosis code(s) for the following: patient suffered a partial traumatic metacarpophalangeal amputation of his right index and middle fingers.

   a. S68.011A, S68.012A

   b. S68.120A, S68.122A

   c. S68.011D, S68.012D

   d. S68.011S

4. Identify the correct ICD-10-PCS code for open thrombectomy, left brachial artery.

   a. R68.89

   b. R79.89

   c. R89.8

   d. R97.2

5. Identify the correct ICD-10-CM diagnosis code(s) for a patient with near-syncope event and nausea.

   a. R55

   b. R55, R11.0

   c. R55, R11.2

   d. R42, R11.0

6. Identify the correct ICD-10-CM diagnosis code(s) for a patient with an elevated glucose tolerance test.

   a. R73.9

   b. R73.01

   c. R73.01, R73.9

   d. R73.02

7. Identify the correct ICD-10-CM diagnosis code(s) for a patient with pneumonia and persistent cough.

    a. R05, J40

    b. J18.9, R05

    c. J18.9

    d. J18.1

8. Identify the correct ICD-10-CM diagnosis code(s) for a patient with seizures; epilepsy ruled out.

    a. R56.9

    b. G40.901

    c. R56.9, G40.909

    d. G40.909

9. Identify the correct ICD-10-CM diagnosis code for a male patient with stress urinary incontinence.

    a. N39.46

    b. R32

    c. N39.3

    d. N39.498

10. Identify the correct ICD-10-CM diagnosis code(s) for a patient hospitalized and treated for vancomycin-resistant sepsis requiring treatment with other special antibiotics.

    a. A49.01

    b. A41.2, Z16.3

    c. A41.9, Z16.21

    d. Z16.3, A41.02

11. Identify the punctuation mark that is used to supplement words or explanatory information that may or may not be present in the statement of a diagnosis in ICD-10-CM coding. The punctuation does not affect the code number assigned to the case and is considered a nonessential modifier.

    a. Parentheses ( )

    b. Square brackets [ ]

    c. Slanted brackets *[ ]*

    d. Braces { }

12. Identify the correct ICD-10-CM diagnosis code(s) for a patient with ST elevated anterolateral wall myocardial infarction.

    a. I21.3

    b. I21.09

    c. I21.4

    d. I21.09, I21.29

13. Identify the correct ICD-10-CM diagnosis code(s) and sequencing for a patient with disseminated candidiasis secondary to AIDS-related complex.

    a. B20, B37.7, Z20.6

    b. B37.7, B20

    c. B20, B37.7, Z21

    d. B20, B37.7

14. Identify the correct ICD-10-CM diagnosis code(s) and proper sequencing for urinary tract infection due to *E. coli*.

    a. N39.0

    b. N39.0, B96.20

    c. B96.20

    d. B96.20, N39.0

15. The 7th character A is used as long as the patient is receiving active treatment for the fracture. When the patient is seen by a new or different provider over the course of treatment for a pathological fracture, assignment of the 7th character is based on _____.

    a. Whether the patient is undergoing active treatment

    b. Whether the provider is seeing the patient for the first time

    c. Whether routine healing will occur

    d. Whether there is a complication in the healing process (i.e., malunion, nonunion, sequelae)

16. Identify the correct ICD-10-CM diagnosis codes for metastatic carcinoma of the colon to the left lung.

    a. C18.9, C34.92

    b. C78.00, C18.9

    c. C18.9, C78.02

    d. C18.9, D49.1

17. Identify the correct ICD-10-CM diagnosis code(s) for a patient with sepsis due to *Staphylococcus aureus*.

    a. A41.01

    b. A41.2

    c. A41.9, B95.61

    d. A41.9

18. Identify the ICD-10-CM diagnosis code(s) for poorly controlled Type 2 diabetes mellitus; mild malnutrition.

    a. E11.65, E46

    b. E10.65, E44.1

    c. E11.65, E44.1

    d. E10.65, E46

19. Identify the ICD-10-CM diagnosis code(s) for neutropenic fever.

    a. D70.9

    b. D70.9, R50.9

    c. D50.81

    d. D70.9, R50.81

20. Time may be considered the key or controlling factor to qualify for a particular level of Evaluation and Management services when _____ percent of the service is _____.

    a. 50 percent; counseling and coordination

    b. 25 percent; examination and counseling

    c. 100 percent; telephone orders

    d. 50 percent; consultation and coordination

21. Category II codes cover all but one of the following topics. Which is *not* addressed by Category II codes?

    a. Patient management

    b. New technology

    c. Therapeutic, preventative, or other interventions

    d. Patient safety

22. Per CPT guidelines, a separate procedure is _____.

    a. Coded when it is performed as part of another, larger procedure

    b. Considered to be an integral part of another, larger service

    c. Never coded under any circumstance

    d. Both a and b

23. CPT was developed and is maintained by _____.

    a. CMS

    b. AMA

    c. Cooperating parties

    d. WHO

24. The codes in the musculoskeletal section of CPT may be used by _____.

    a. Orthopedic surgeons only

    b. Orthopedic surgeons and emergency department physicians

    c. Any physician

    d. Orthopedic surgeons and neurosurgeons

25. Observation E/M codes (99218–99220) are used in physician billing when _____.

    a. A patient is admitted and discharged on the same date

    b. A patient is admitted for routine nursing care following surgery

    c. A patient does not meet admission criteria

    d. A patient is referred to a designated observation status

26. Documentation in the history of use of drugs, alcohol, and tobacco is considered as part of the _____.

    a. Past medical history

    b. Social history

    c. Systems review

    d. History of present illness

27. Tissue transplanted from one individual to another of the same species, but different genotype is called a(n) _____.

    a. Autograft

    b. Xenograft

    c. Allograft or allogeneic graft

    d. Heterograft

28. Mohs micrographic surgery involves the surgeon acting as _____.

    a. Both plastic surgeon and general surgeon

    b. Both surgeon and pathologist

    c. Both plastic surgeon and dermatologist

    d. Both dermatologist and pathologist

29. If an orthopedic surgeon attempted to reduce a fracture but was unsuccessful in obtaining acceptable alignment, what type of code should be assigned for the procedure?

    a. A "with manipulation" code

    b. A "without manipulation" code

    c. An unlisted procedure code

    d. An E/M code only

30. Discharge services provided to a normal newborn, admitted and discharged on the same day, is coded _____.

    a. 99238

    b. 99460

    c. 99239

    d. 99463

31. In coding arterial catheterizations, when the tip of the catheter is manipulated from the insertion into the aorta and then out into another artery, this is called _____.

    a. Selective catheterization

    b. Nonselective catheterization

    c. Manipulative catheterization

    d. Radical catheterization

32. When coding a selective catheterization in CPT, how are codes assigned?

    a. Include introduction and all lesser order selective catheterizations used in the approach

    b. Always assign an add-on code to report placement and technical components

    c. Do not include local anesthesia or diagnostic imaging

    d. Use the first order or higher catheterization within the vascular families supplied by the first order vessel

Domain 2   *Reimbursement Methodologies*

33. How does Medicare or other third-party payers determine whether the patient has medical necessity for the tests, procedures, or treatment billed on a claim form?

    a. By requesting the medical record for each service provided

    b. By reviewing all the diagnosis codes assigned to explain the reasons the services were provided

    c. By reviewing all physician orders

    d. By reviewing the discharge summary and history and physical report of the patient over the last year

34. What is the name of the organization that develops the billing form that hospitals are required to use?

    a. American Academy of Billing Forms (AABF)

    b. National Uniform Billing Committee (NUBC)

    c. National Uniform Claims Committee (NUCC)

    d. American Billing and Claims Academy (ABCA)

35. What healthcare organizations collect UHDDS data?

    a. All outpatient settings including physician clinics and ambulatory surgical centers

    b. All outpatient settings including cancer centers, independent testing facilities, and nursing homes

    c. All non outpatient settings including acute care, short-term care, long-term care, and psychiatric hospitals; home health agencies; rehabilitation facilities; and nursing homes

    d. All inpatient settings and outpatient settings with a focus on ambulatory surgical centers

36. What was the goal of the MS-DRG system?

    a. To improve Medicare's capability to recognize severity of illness in its inpatient hospital payments. The new system is projected to increase payments to hospitals for services provided to sicker patients and decrease payments for treating less severely ill patients.

    b. To improve Medicare's capability to recognize poor quality of care and pay hospitals on an incentive grid that allows hospitals to be paid by performance.

    c. To improve Medicare's capability to recognize groups of data by patient populations, which will further allow Medicare to adjust the hospitals' wage indexes based on the data. This adjustment will be a system to pay hospitals fairly across all geographic locations.

    d. To improve Medicare's capability to recognize practice patterns among hospitals that are inappropriately optimizing payments by keeping patients in the hospital longer than the median length of stay.

37. What is the basic formula for calculating each MS-DRG hospital payment?

    a. Hospital payment = DRG relative weight × hospital base rate

    b. Hospital payment = DRG relative weight × hospital base rate − 1

    c. Hospital payment = DRG relative weight / hospital base rate + 1

    d. Hospital payment = DRG relative weight / hospital base rate

38. What are the possible "add-on" payments that a hospital could receive in addition to the basic Medicare DRG payment?

    a. Additional payments may be made for locum tenens, increased emergency room services, stays over the average length of stay, and cost outlier cases.

    b. Additional payments may be made to critical access hospitals, for higher-than-normal volumes, unexpected hospital emergencies, and cost outlier cases.

    c. Additional payments may be made for increased emergency room services, critical access hospitals, increased labor costs, and cost outlier cases.

    d. Additional payments may be made to disproportionate share hospitals for indirect medical education, new technologies, and cost outlier cases.

39. What is the name of the national program to detect and correct improper payments in the Medicare Fee-for-Service (FFS) program?

    a. Medicare administrative contractors (MACs)

    b. Recovery audit contractors (RACs)

    c. Comprehensive error rate testing (CERT)

    d. Fiscal intermediaries (FIs)

40. The middle process of the revenue cycle's objectives is _____.

    a. Manage clinical procedural documentation and charging services

    b. Denial and appeal management

    c. Revenue audits and recovery procedures

    d. Registration processing and quality audits

41. Which answer is *not* required for assignment of the MS-DRG?

    a. Diagnoses and procedures (principal and secondary)

    b. Attending and consulting physicians

    c. Presence of major or other complications and comorbidities (MCC or CC)

    d. Discharge disposition or status

42. What is the maximum number of diagnosis codes that can appear on the UB-04 paper claim form locator 67 for a hospital inpatient principal and secondary diagnoses?

    a. 35

    b. 25

    c. 18

    d. 9

43. Which of the following situations would be identified by the NCCI edits?

    a. Determining the MS-DRG

    b. Billing for two services that are prohibited from being billed on the same day

    c. Whether data submitted electronically were successfully submitted

    d. Receiving the remittance advice

44. A hospital needs to know how much Medicare paid on a claim so they can bill the secondary insurance. What should the hospital refer to?

    a. Explanation of benefits

    b. Medicare Summary Notice

    c. Remittance advice

    d. Coordination of benefits

45. A patient has two health insurance policies: Medicare and a Medicare supplement. Which of the following statements is true?

    a. The patient receives any monies paid by the insurance companies over and above the charges.

    b. Monies paid to the healthcare provider cannot exceed charges.

    c. The decision on which company is primary is based on remittance advice.

    d. The patient should not have a Medicare supplement.

46. The purpose of a physician query is to _____.

    a. Identify the MS-DRG

    b. Identify the principal diagnosis

    c. Improve documentation for patient care and proper reimbursement

    d. Increase reimbursement as form of optimization

47. What is the term used when a Medicare hospital inpatient admission results in exceptionally high costs when compared to other cases in the same DRG?

    a. Rate increase

    b. Charge outlier

    c. Cost outlier

    d. Day outlier

48. What is a chargemaster?

    a. Cost-sharing in which the policy or certificate holder pays a preestablished percentage of eligible expenses after the deductible has been met

    b. A plan that converts the organization's goals and objectives into targets for revenue and spending

    c. A financial management system that contains information about the organization's charges for the healthcare services it provides to patients

    d. Charged amounts that are billed as costs by an organization to the current year's activities of operation

49. A fee schedule is _____.

    a. Developed by third-party payers and includes a list of healthcare services, procedures, and charges associated with each

    b. Developed by providers and includes a list of healthcare services, procedures, and charges associated with each

    c. Developed by third-party payers and includes a list of healthcare services provided to a patient

    d. Developed by providers and lists charge codes

50. The charge description master contains all of the following general data elements except:

    a. Charge code description

    b. DRG assignment

    c. Insurance coverage determination

    d. Price

51. If a provider believes a service may be denied by Medicare because it could be considered unnecessary, the provider must notify the patient before the treatment begins by using a(n) _____.

    a. Advance beneficiary notice (ABN)

    b. Advance notice of coverage (ANC)

    c. Notice of payment (NOP)

    d. Consent for payment (CFP)

52. Assignment of benefits is a contract between a physician and Medicare in which the physician agrees to bill Medicare directly for covered services and the beneficiary for _____ and to accept the Medicare payment as payment in full.

    a. Coinsurance or deductible

    b. Deductible only

    c. Coinsurance only

    d. Balance of charges

53. A provision of the law that established the resource-based relative value scale (RBRVS) stipulates that refinements to relative value units (RVUs) must maintain _____.

    a. Moderate rate increases

    b. Market basket increases

    c. Budget neutrality

    d. Sustainable growth rate

54. Reimbursement for healthcare services is dependent on patients having a(n) _____.

    a. Attending physician

    b. Insurance benefit

    c. Explanation of benefits

    d. Qualified provider

55. Health insurance for spouses, children, or both is known as _____.

    a. Dependent (family) coverage

    b. Individual (single) coverage

    c. Group coverage

    d. Inclusive coverage

Domain 3   *Health Records and Data Content*

56. Documentation regarding a patient's marital status; dietary, sleep, and exercise patterns; and use of coffee, tobacco, alcohol, and other drugs may be found in the:

    a. Physical examination record

    b. History record

    c. Operative report

    d. Radiological report

57. A patient with known COPD and hypertension under treatment was admitted to the hospital with symptoms of a lower abdominal pain. He undergoes a laparoscopic appendectomy and develops a fever. The patient was subsequently discharged from the hospital with a principal diagnosis of acute appendicitis and secondary diagnoses of postoperative infection, COPD, and hypertension. Which of the following diagnoses should *not* be tagged as POA?

    a. Postoperative infection

    b. Appendicitis

    c. COPD

    d. Hypertension

58. Which of the following would *not* be found in a medical history?

    a. Chief complaint

    b. Vital signs

    c. Present illness

    d. Review of systems

59. Which of the following reports includes names of the surgeon and assistants, date, duration and description of the procedure, and any specimens removed?

    a. Operative report

    b. Anesthesia report

    c. Pathology report

    d. Laboratory report

60. The Joint Commission and CMS require hospitals to inform families of the opportunity to donate organs, tissue, or eyes. The name of the criteria that potential donors must meet is _____.

    a. United Network of Organ Sharing (UNOS)

    b. Conditions of Participation

    c. Personal Health Record (PHR)

    d. Do Not Resuscitate (DNR)

61. Identify the acute-care record report where the following information would be found:

    Gross Description: Received fresh designated left lacrimal gland is a single, unoriented, irregular, tan-pink portion of soft tissue measuring $0.8 \times 0.6 \times 0.1$ cm, which is submitted entirely intact in one cassette.

    a. Medical history

    b. Medical laboratory report

    c. Pathology report

    d. Physical examination

62. Which organization developed the first hospital standardization program?

    a. Joint Commission

    b. American Osteopathic Association

    c. American College of Surgeons

    d. American Association of Medical Colleges

63. The hospital is revising its policy on medical record documentation. Currently, all entries in the medical record must be legible, complete, dated, and signed. The committee chairperson wants to add that, in addition, all entries must have the time noted. However, another clinician suggests that adding the time of notation is difficult and rarely may be correct since personal watches and hospital clocks may not be coordinated. Another committee member agrees and says only electronic documentation needs a time stamp. Given this discussion, which of the following might the HIM director suggest?

    a. Suggest that only hospital clock time be noted in clinical documentation

    b. Suggest that only electronic documentation have time noted

    c. Inform the committee that according to the Medicare Conditions of Participation, all documentation must be authenticated and dated

    d. Inform the committee that according to the Medicare Conditions of Participation, only medication orders must include date and time

64. When correcting erroneous information in a health record, which of the following is *not* appropriate?

    a. Print "error" above the entry

    b. Enter the correction in chronological sequence

    c. Add the reason for the change

    d. Use black pen to obliterate the entry

65. Within the ambulatory care setting, the Joint Commission requires that ambulatory patients have certain documentation present in their record by the third visit. The _____ has additional requirements for the content of the ambulatory record.

    a. EMTALA

    b. AAAHC

    c. CMS

    d. Patient's provider

66. In a routine health record quantitative analysis review, it was found that a physician dictated a discharge summary on 1/26/20XX. The patient, however, was discharged two days later. In this case, what would be the best course of action?

    a. Request that the physician dictate another discharge summary.

    b. Have the record analyst note the date discrepancy.

    c. Request the physician dictate an addendum to the discharge summary.

    d. File the record as complete because the discharge summary includes all of the pertinent patient information.

67. During an audit of health records, the HIM director finds that transcribed reports are being changed by the author up to a week after initial transcription. The director is concerned that changes occurring this long after transcription jeopardize the legal principle that documentation must occur near the time of the event. To remedy this situation, the HIM director should recommend which of the following?

    a. Immediately stop the practice of changing transcribed reports.

    b. Develop a facility policy that defines the acceptable period of time allowed for a transcribed document to remain in draft form.

    c. Conduct a verification audit.

    d. Alert hospital legal counsel of the practice.

68. During a review of documentation practices, the HIM director finds that nurses are routinely using the copy-and-paste function of the hospital's new EHR system for documenting nursing notes. In some cases, nurses are copying and pasting the objective data from the lab system and intake–output records as well as the patient's subjective complaints and symptoms originally documented by another practitioner. Which of the following should the HIM director do to ensure the nurses are following acceptable documentation practices?

    a. Inform the nurses that "copy and paste" is not acceptable and to stop this practice immediately.

    b. Determine how many nurses are involved in this practice.

    c. Institute an in-service training session on documentation practices.

    d. Develop policies and procedures related to cutting, copying, and pasting documentation in the EHR system.

69. Who is responsible for writing and signing discharge summaries and discharge instructions?

    a. Attending physician

    b. Head nurse

    c. Primary physician

    d. Admitting nurse

70. Where would a coder who needed to locate the histology of a tissue sample most likely find this information?

    a. Pathology report

    b. Progress notes

    c. Nurse's notes

    d. Operative report

Domain 4 *Compliance*

71. An HIM professional's ethical obligations _____.

    a. Apply regardless of employment site

    b. Are limited to the employer

    c. Apply to only the patient

    d. Are limited to the employer and patient

72. Which of the following is the concept of the right of an individual to be left alone?

    a. Privacy

    b. Bioethics

    c. Security

    d. Confidentiality

73. What should be done when the HIM department's error or accuracy rate is deemed unacceptable?

    a. A corrective action should be taken.

    b. The problem should be treated as an isolated incident.

    c. The formula for determining the rate may need to be adjusted.

    d. Re-audit the problem area.

74. Statements that define the performance expectations and structures or processes that must be in place are _____.

    a. Rules

    b. Policies

    c. Guidelines

    d. Standards

75. A coding compliance program should contain the same components as the organization's:

    a. Quality improvement process

    b. HIPAA rules

    c. Compliance plan

    d. Governing Board policies

76. How are amendments handled in an EHR?

    a. Automatically appended to the original note; no additional signature is required.

    b. Amendments must be entered by the same person as the original note.

    c. Amendments cannot be entered after 24 hours of the event's occurrence.

    d. The amendment must have a separate signature, date, and time.

77. The Privacy Rule establishes that a patient has the right of access to inspect and obtain a copy of his or her PHI _____.

    a. For as long as it is maintained

    b. For six years

    c. Forever

    d. For 12 months

78. HIPAA regulations _____.

    a. Never preempt state statutes

    b. Always preempt state statutes

    c. Preempt less-strict state statutes where they exist

    d. Preempt stricter state statutes where they exist

79. The Privacy Rule applies to _____.

    a. All covered entities involved with transmitting or performing any electronic transactions specified in the act

    b. Healthcare providers only

    c. Only healthcare providers that receive Medicare reimbursement

    d. Only entities funded by the federal government

80. Which of the following is the area responsible for limiting disclosure of private matters including the responsibility to use, disclose, or release such information only with the knowledge and consent of the individual?

    a. Privacy

    b. Bioethics

    c. Security

    d. Confidentiality

81. Which of the following is *not* an accepted accrediting body for behavioral healthcare organizations?

    a. American Psychological Association

    b. Joint Commission

    c. Commission on Accreditation of Rehabilitation Facilities

    d. National Committee for Quality Assurance

82. Which of the following is an example of a unique identifier for an individual heath record to ensure that the information in the record is not misplaced, lost, or confused with information for another person each time a patient visits a facility?

    a. Account number

    b. Health record number

    c. Admission date

    d. Discharge date

83. What type of organization works under contract with the CMS to conduct Medicare and Medicaid certification surveys for hospitals?

    a. Accreditation organizations

    b. Certification organizations

    c. State licensure agencies

    d. Conditions of participation agencies

84. Which of the following threatens the "need-to-know" principle?

    a. Backdating progress notes

    b. Blanket authorization

    c. HIPAA regulations

    d. Surgical consent

Domain 5   *Information Technologies*

85. A hospital is planning on allowing coding professionals to work at home. The hospital is in the process of identifying strategies to minimize the security risks associated with this practice. Which of the following would be *best* to ensure that data breaches are minimized when the home computer is unattended?

    a. User name and password

    b. Automatic session terminations

    c. Cable locks

    d. Encryption

86. A coding analyst consistently enters the wrong code for patient gender in the electronic billing system. What data quality or data integrity measures should be in place to ensure that only allowable code numbers are entered?

    a. Access controls

    b. Audit trail

    c. Edit checks

    d. Password controls

87. Which of the following would be the *best* technique to ensure that registration clerks consistently use the correct notation for assigning admission date in an electronic health record (EHR)?

    a. Make admission date a required field

    b. Provide an input mask for entering data in the field

    c. Make admission date a numeric field

    d. Provide sufficient space for input of data

88. In hospitals, automated systems for registering patients and tracking their encounters are commonly known as _____ systems.

    a. MIS

    b. CDS

    c. R-ADT

    d. ABC

89. Which of the following provides organizations with the ability to access data from multiple databases and to combine the results into a single questions-and-reporting interface?

    a. Client-server computer

    b. Data warehouse

    c. Local area network

    d. Internet

90. The _____ hospital system captures demographic and insurance data, supplies the data to other applications and tracks patients:

    a. Patient financial system (PFSC)

    b. Registration-admission-discharge-transfer (R-ADT)

    c. Revenue Cycle management (RCM)

    d. Clinical Data Repository (CDR)

91. A(n) _____ is computer software that assists in determining coding accuracy and reliability.

    a. Encoder

    b. Interface

    c. Diagnosis-related group

    d. Record locator service

92. The _____ uses expert or artificial intelligence software to automatically assign code numbers.

    a. Functional EHR

    b. NHIN

    c. NLP encoding system

    d. Grouper

Domain 6 *Confidentiality and Privacy*

93. All states have laws that require _____.

    a. Disclosure of health information, even if patient authorizes it

    b. Reporting of births and deaths

    c. Reporting of suspected child abuse or neglect

    d. All of the above

94. Which of the following ethical principles is being followed when an HIT professional ensures that patient information is only released to those who have a legal right to access it?

    a. Autonomy

    b. Beneficence

    c. Justice

    d. Nonmaleficence

95. Which of the following is a threat to data security?

    a. Encryption

    b. People

    c. Red flags

    d. Access controls

96. Under the HIPAA privacy standard, which of the following types of protected health information (PHI) must be specifically identified in an authorization?

    a. History and physical reports

    b. Operative reports

    c. Consultation reports

    d. Psychotherapy notes

97. What penalties can be enforced against a person or entity that willfully and knowingly violates the HIPAA Privacy Rule with the intent to sell, transfer, or use PHI for commercial advantage, personal gain, or malicious harm?

    a. A fine of not more than $10,000 only

    b. A fine of not more than $10,000, not more than one year in jail, or both

    c. A fine of not more than $5,000 only

    d. A fine of not more than $250,000, not more than 10 years in jail, or both

98. An HIT, using her password, can access and change data in the hospital's master patient index. A billing clerk, using his password, cannot perform the same function. Limiting the class of information and functions that can be performed by these two employees is managed by _____.

    a. Network controls

    b. Audit trails

    c. Administrative controls

    d. Access controls

99. An employee in the physical therapy department arrives early every morning to snoop through the clinical information system for potential information about neighbors and friends. What security mechanisms should be implemented to prevent this security breach?

    a. Audit controls

    b. Information access controls

    c. Facility access controls

    d. Workstation security

100. What should a hospital do when a state law requires more stringent privacy protection than the federal HIPAA privacy standard?

    a. Ignore the state law and follow the HIPAA standard

    b. Follow the state law and ignore the HIPAA standard

    c. Comply with both the state law and the HIPAA standard

    d. Ignore both the state law and the HIPAA standard and follow relevant accreditation standards

ANSWER KEY

CCA Practice Questions

1. a   Index Carcinoma, in situ, see also Neoplasm, by site, in situ (Schraffenberger 2018, 137, 145).

2. b   Index Melanoma (malignant), shoulder. Melanoma is considered a malignant neoplasm and is referenced as such in the index of ICD-10-CM. The term "benign neoplasm" is considered a growth that does not invade adjacent structures or spread to distant sites but may displace or exert pressure on adjacent structures (Schraffenberger 2018, 137, 145).

3. b   CMS is responsible for updating the procedure classification (ICD-10-PCS) (Giannangelo 2016, 124).

4. c   "Causal condition first" general coding guideline states, "this code may be assigned as principal diagnosis when the causal condition is unknown or not specified." (CMS, CG7, 2019).

5. d   The seventh character provides information about encounter of care, such as initial encounter, subsequent encounter, or sequelae (Giannangelo 2016, 123).

6. c   The fourth character captures etiology. The fifth captures anatomic site. The sixth captures severity (Giannangelo 2016, 123).

7. a   Codes must be at least three characters, with a decimal point used after the third character (Giannangelo 2016, 123).

8. b   When a note appears under a three-character code in ICD-10-CM, it applies to all codes within that category (Giannangelo 2016, 123).

9. d   ICD-10-CM includes diagnoses only. In the development of the ICD-10 code sets, it was determined that creating a separate volume for procedures would be insufficient. Because of this, an entirely new procedure code system, ICD-10-PCS, was developed (Giannangelo 2016, 123).

10. a   Coding Guideline I.A.12.a explicitly states this exception (CMS 2018a).

11. a   Index Adenoma, adrenal (cortex). Index Syndrome, Conn's. According to the Index in ICD-10-CM, except where otherwise indicated, the morphological varieties of adenoma should be coded by site as for "Neoplasm, benign" (Schraffenberger 2018, 146–147).

12. a   CPT is a comprehensive descriptive listing of terms and codes for reporting diagnostic and therapeutic procedures and medical services (Giannangelo 2016, 119).

13. c   Index Contusion, cerebral. Add a sixth character of "1" for loss of consciousness of 30 minutes or less. Cerebral contusions are often caused by a blow to the head. A cerebral contusion is a more severe injury involving a bruise of the brain with bleeding into the brain tissue, but without disruption of the brain's continuity. The loss of consciousness that occurs often lasts longer than that of a concussion. Codes for cerebral laceration and contusion range from S06.0–S06.9 with sixth characters indicating whether a loss of consciousness or concussion occurred (Schraffenberger 2018, 581–582).

14. d   The code selection is determined by measuring the greatest clinical diameter of the apparent lesion plus that margin required for complete excision (lesion diameter plus the most narrow margins required equals the excised diameter) (AMA 2018, 99).

15. c   Complex closure includes the repair of wounds requiring more than layered closure, namely, scar revision, debridement, extensive undermining, stents, or retention sutures (AMA 2018, 90).

16. a   Guideline I.C.15.q.2 Retained Products of Conception following an abortion: Subsequent admissions for retained products of conception following a spontaneous or legally induced abortion are assigned the appropriate code from category O03, spontaneous abortion, or codes O07.4, Failed attempted termination of pregnancy without complication and Z33.2, Encounter for elective termination of pregnancy. This advice is appropriate even when the patient was discharged previously with a discharge diagnosis of complete abortion (Schraffenberger 2018, 481–482).

17. c   The term "urosepsis" is a nonspecific term and is not codable in ICD-10-CM. It is not to be considered synonymous with sepsis. It has no default code in the Alphabetic Index. Should a provider use this term, he or she must be queried for clarification (Schraffenberger 2018, 114).

18. c   Guideline I.C.2.a If treatment is directed at the malignancy, designate the malignancy as the principal diagnosis. The only exception to this guideline is if a patient admission or encounter is solely for the administration of chemotherapy, immunotherapy, or radiation therapy, assign the appropriate Z51.-code as the first-listed or principal diagnosis and the diagnosis or problem for which the service is being performed as a secondary diagnosis (Schraffenberger 2018, 139).

19. b   Gastroenteritis is characterized by diarrhea, nausea, and vomiting, and abdominal cramps. Codes for symptoms, signs, and ill-defined conditions from Chapter 18 of the ICD-10-CM codebook are not to be used as the principal diagnosis when a related definitive diagnosis has been established. Patients can have several chronic conditions that coexist at the time of their hospital admission and qualify as additional diagnosis such as COPD and angina (Schraffenberger 2018, 547–549).

20. c   In this circumstance, both codes F45.8 and G47.63 can be coded together because psychogenic dysmenorrhea is also an inclusion term; patient could have both conditions (CMS 2018a).

21. a   In the unusual instance when two or more diagnoses equally meet the criteria for principal diagnosis, as determined by the circumstances of admission, diagnostic workup, and the therapy provided, and the Alphabetic Index, Tabular List, or another coding guideline does not provide sequencing direction in such cases, any one of the diagnoses may be sequenced first (Schraffenberger 2018, 93–94).

22. c   For reporting purposes the definition for "other diagnoses" is interpreted as additional conditions that affect patient care in terms of requiring: clinical evaluation, therapeutic treatment, diagnostic procedures, extended length of hospital stay, increased nursing care, and monitoring (Schraffenberger 2018, 98–99).

23. c   A patient in status asthmaticus fails to respond to therapy administered during an asthmatic attack. This is a life-threatening condition that requires emergency care and likely hospitalization (Schraffenberger 2018, 347).

24. d   Signs, symptoms, abnormal test results, or other reasons for the outpatient visit are used when a physician qualifies a diagnostic statement as "rule out" or other similar terms indicating uncertainty. In the outpatient setting the condition qualified in that statement should not be coded as if it existed. Rather, the condition should be coded to the highest degree of certainty, such as the sign or symptom the patient exhibits. In this case, assign the code R07.9 Chest pain, unspecified (Schraffenberger 2018, 103; Coding Guidelines Section IV.H.).

25. c   For outpatient encounters for diagnostic tests that have been interpreted by a physician, and the final report is available at the time of coding, code any confirmed or definitive diagnosis(es) documented in the interpretation. Do not code related signs and symptoms as additional diagnosis. Note: This differs from the coding practice in the hospital inpatient setting regarding abnormal findings on test results (Schraffenberger 2018, 103).

26. c   The disproportion was specified as cephalopelvic; thus the correct ICD-10-CM code is O65.4. Two codes are required for anesthesia: one for the planned vaginal delivery (01967) and an add-on code (01968) to describe anesthesia for cesarean delivery following planned vaginal delivery converted to cesarean. An instructional note guides the coder to use 01968 with 01967 (AMA 2018, 68).

27. d   CMS designed ICD-10-PCS with goals to improve coding accuracy, reduce training effort, and improve communication with physicians. It is not used to collect data about nursing care (Giannangelo 2016, 124).

28. d   Additional signs and symptoms that may not be associated with a disease process should be coded when present (Schraffenberger, 2018, 36).

29. a   Partial nephrectomy is an example of the root procedure Excision. A portion of the body part is cut out or off, without replacement (Giannangelo, 125).

30. b   The assignment of a diagnosis code is based on the provider's diagnostic statement that the condition exists (CMS 2018).

31. b   Code I63.50 is assigned when the diagnosis states stroke, cerebrovascular, or cerebrovascular accident (CVA) without further specification. In this case, the patient had an occlusion without a stroke. Code I66.9 is assigned. The health record should be reviewed to make sure nothing more specific is available. Conditions resulting from an acute cerebrovascular disease, such as aphasia or hemiplegia, should be coded as well. The side that the hemiparesis is affecting is not stated, so code G81.90 is assigned (Schraffenberger 2018, 317–319).

32. a   Acute respiratory failure, code J96.00–J96.02, may be assigned as a principal or secondary diagnosis depending on the circumstances of the inpatient admission. Chapter-specific coding guidelines (obstetrics, poisoning, HIV, newborn) provide specific sequencing direction. Because the respiratory failure occurred after admission, it is listed as a secondary diagnosis and the congestive heart failure is listed first (Schraffenberger 2018, 350–351).

33. d   Guideline I.C.19.e.5(a) Adverse effects can occur in situations in which medication is administered properly and prescribed correctly in both therapeutic and diagnostic procedures. An adverse effect can occur when everything is done correctly. The first-listed diagnosis is the manifestation or the nature of the adverse effect, such as the hematuria. Locate the drug in the Substance column of the Table of Drugs and Chemicals in the Alphabetic Index to Diseases. Assign the appropriate seventh character to the drug or chemical code to identify whether the healthcare was provided during the initial encounter, a subsequent encounter, or for a sequel (Schraffenberger 2018, 600).

34. c   Guideline I.C.9.e.1 for encounters occurring while the myocardial infarction is equal to, or less than, four weeks old, including transfers to another acute setting or a postacute setting, and the patient requires continued care for the myocardial infarction, codes form category I21 may continue to be reported (Schraffenberger 2018, 305–306).

35. b   The principal diagnosis determines the MDC assignment (Giannangelo 2016, 134).

36. a   All claims involving inpatient admissions to general acute care hospitals or other facilities that are subject to law or regulation mandating collection of present on admission information. *Present on admission* (POA) is defined as present at the time the order for inpatient admission occurs. Conditions that develop during an outpatient encounter, including emergency department, observation, or outpatient surgery, are considered POA. Any condition that occurs after admission is not considered a POA condition (Schraffenberger 2018, 95).

37. b   A *complication* is a secondary condition that arises during hospitalization and is thought to increase the length of stay by at least one day for approximately 75 percent of the patients (Gordon and Gordon 2016a, 441).

38. b   *Sepsis* refers to a systemic immune response associated with the presence of pathological microorganisms or toxins in the blood, which can include bacteria, viruses, fungi, or other organisms. Code A41.01 is assigned for sepsis due to *Staphylococcus aureus*. Because abdominal pain is a symptom of diverticulitis, only the diverticulitis of the colon, unspecified part of colon, K57.92 is coded. Per Guideline I.C.1.d.4, if the reason for admission is both sepsis…and a localized infection…a code for the underlying systemic infection (sepsis) should be assigned first and the code for the localized infection (diverticulitis) should be assigned as a secondary diagnosis (Schraffenberger 2018, 120–121).

39. c   Guideline I.C.2.d Primary malignancy previously excised is coded to category Z85, Personal history of malignancy neoplasm if there is no further treatment directed to that site and there is no evidence of any existing primary malignancy. Because the malignancy recurred, it is coded as a current malignancy, code C67.3, and no Z code is included (Schraffenberger 2018, 140).

40. a   The physician or other qualified healthcare practitioner who is legally accountable for establishing the patient's diagnosis is acceptable because this information is typically documented by other clinicians involved in the patient's care (CMS 2018b).

41. d   *Z codes* are diagnosis codes and indicate a reason for healthcare encounter (Schraffenberger 2018, 646–647).

42. b   The fracture is the principal diagnosis, with the contusions as a secondary diagnosis. The fracture is what required the most treatment. Procedures for the reduction, debridement, need to be coded (Schraffenberger 2018, 92, 574–578).

43. d   Begin with the main term Repositioning; electrode, heart (Kuehn 2019, 272–273).

44. a   Code 54065 is correct because the physician determines that the destruction, by any method, is extensive (Kuehn 2019, 169).

45. d   Modifier −24 is used for unrelated evaluation and management service by the same physician during a postoperative period (Kuehn 2019, 55).

46. d   One code is assigned for alcohol dependence with alcohol withdrawal. Alcohol abuse is not assigned per Excludes 1 note under F10.1. Under F10, the "use additional code" note for blood alcohol level (Y90.-) applies to this case since blood alcohol level is documented (Schraffenberger 2018, 202, 207–210).

47. a   The anemia would be sequenced first based on principal diagnosis guidelines. Since the anemia is not specified as "acute blood loss," it's coded to "chronic blood loss" because "chronic" is a nonessential modifier for "blood loss anemia" (Schraffenberger 2018, 93, 163–169).

48. d   The patient was admitted for the senile cortical cataract and the procedures were completed for that condition. This follows the UHDDS guidelines for principal diagnosis selection. Per coding guidelines, there is an assumed causal relationship given between the Type 2 diabetes and the cataract, so E11.36 would be correct (CMS 2018).

49. d   The patient was admitted and COPD is listed as the principal diagnosis. Code J44.1 is used when the medical record includes documentation of COPD with acute exacerbation. ICD-10-CM presumes a cause-and-effect relationship and classifies chronic kidney disease with hypertension as hypertensive chronic kidney disease, code I12.9; however, the code also at category I12 directs the coder to also code the chronic renal failure N18.9 (Schraffenberger 2018, 92–97, 301).

50. a   Code only confirmed cases. Confirmation does not require documentation of the type of test performed according to the Coding Guideline I.C.1.f (CMS 2018a).

51. c   A bronchoscopy with brushings and washings is considered a diagnostic bronchoscopy and not a biopsy. Code 31623 specifies brushings, and code 31622 is selected for washings (Kuehn 2019, 113).

52. d   Modifiers are appended to the code to provide more information or to alert the payer that a payment change is required. Modifier −55 is used to identify the physician provided only postoperative care services for a particular procedure (Kuehn 2019, 57).

53. b   Index main term: Destruction, hemorrhoid, thermal. Thermal includes infrared coagulation (Kuehn 2019, 149).

54. c   A *logic-based encoder* prompts the user through a variety of questions and choices based on the clinical terminology entered. The coder selects the most accurate code for a service or condition and any possible complications or comorbidities (Sayles 2016, 74–75).

55. a   Index main term: Depression; then index subterm: major, recurrent, see disorder, depressive, recurrent. The index gives the following in the cross reference: Disorder, depressive, recurrent, current episode, severe (without mention of psychotic symptoms) F33.2 (Schraffenberger 2018, 26–27).

56. c   Main term for procedure: Excision; subterm: esophagus, upper (Schraffenberger 2018, 42–44).

57. d   Codes for symptoms, signs, and ill-defined conditions are not to be used as the principal diagnosis when a related definitive diagnosis has been established. The flank pain would not be coded because it is a symptom of the calculus. Root operation Dilation is coded because the intent is to expand the lumen of the tubular body part, the ureters. The stent is the device that is reported in character 6. One code is assigned for "bilateral" instead of two codes, indication "left, right" when a "bilateral" option is available (Schraffenberger 2018, 51, 93).

58. c Main term for diagnosis: Incontinence; subterm: stress. Common procedural term: Suspension; subterm: urethra, see Reposition, Urinary System, table 0TS (Schraffenberger 2018, 8, 50–52).

59. c Index the main term of Hernia repair; inguinal; incarcerated. The age of the patient and the fact that the hernia is not recurrent make the choice 49507 (Kuehn 2019, 151–153).

60. b Coding Guideline I.C.4.a.3 states that if the documentation identifies that the patient uses insulin but not the type of diabetes, the code assignment is E11.

61. b Main term of Hysteroscopy; lysis; adhesions (Kuehn 2019, 173).

62. d In the abdomen, peritoneum, and omentum subsection, the exploratory laparotomy is a separate procedure and should not be reported when it is part of a larger procedure. The code of 49000 is not reported because laparotomy is the approach to the surgery. The code 58720 includes bilateral so the modifier −50 is not necessary to report (Kuehn 2019, 151–152).

63. c Dialysis, end-stage renal disease. Code 90966 is for end-stage renal disease (ESRD)-related services for home dialysis per full month for patients 20 years and older (Smith 2019, 263).

64. c Code 97113, Therapeutic procedure, one or more areas, each 15 minutes of aquatic therapy with therapeutic exercises, is billable per 15 minutes of therapy. The patient was treated for 30 minutes; therefore, code 97113 should be reported twice. Modifier −50 is not applicable because the service is not a bilateral procedure (AMA 2018, 729).

65. a The *geometric mean LOS* is defined as the total days of service, excluding any outliers or transfers, divided by the total number of patients (Hazelwood and Venable 2016, 224).

66. b Multiple surgical procedures with payment status indicator T performed during the same operative session are discounted. The highest-weighted procedure is fully reimbursed. All other procedures with payment status indicator T are reimbursed at 50 percent (Casto and Forrestal 2015, 182).

67. a There are not LCDs and NDCs for every type of procedure or service that could be provided for a patient (Malmgren and Solberg 2016, 243).

68. a Psychiatric and rehabilitation hospitals, long-term care hospitals, children's hospitals, cancer hospitals, and critical access hospitals are paid on the basis of reasonable cost, subject to payment limits per discharge or under separate PPS (Gordon and Gordon 2016a, 440).

69. c Diagnosis-related groupings (DRGs) are classified by one of 25 major diagnostic categories (MDCs) (Hazelwood and Venable 2016, 224).

70. a Medicare Part A is generally provided free of charge to individuals age 65 and over who are eligible for Social Security. The coverage is provided to those with end-stage renal disease (Hazelwood and Venable 2016, 206).

71. b Critical access hospitals are paid on a cost-based payment system and are not part of the prospective payment system (Kellogg 2016a, 32).

72. a Third-party payers who reimburse providers on a fee-for-service basis generally update fee schedules on an annual basis (Gordon and Gordon 2016a, 421).

73. a   Physicians submit claims via the electronic format (screen 837P), which takes the place of the CMS-1500 billing form (Gordon and Gordon 2016a, 422).

74. b   To accept assignment means the provider or supplier accepts, as payment in full, the allowed charge based on the fee schedule (Gordon and Gordon 2016a, 427).

75. c   Review the elements of the hospital compliance program with the employee (Prater 2016, 557).

76. b   Since 1983, the prospective payment systems have been used to manage the costs of the Medicare and Medicaid programs (Gordon and Gordon 2016a, 440).

77. c   Access to an indwelling IV or insertion of a subcutaneous catheter or port for the purpose of a therapeutic infusion is considered part of the procedure and not separately billed (Smith 2019, 276–278).

78. a   The goal of a compliance program is to reduce the liability with regards to fraud and abuse (Foltz et al. 2016, 457).

79. a   Any secondary diagnoses assigned present on admission status will have a negative impact on reimbursement if no other code on the claim is assigned as a complication or comorbidity or a major complication or comorbidity (Russo 2010, 30).

80. c   Payment for separately paid APCs depends on the status indicator assigned to each HCPCS code. This particular example allows separate payment on all five codes based on separately paid status indicator assignment (Hazelwood and Venable 2016, 228–229).

81. c   Out-of-pocket expenses are the healthcare expenses that the insured party is responsible for paying after the insurer has paid its amount. In the example, after the allowed charges of 80%, or $400, are covered by the insurance company, the patient will be responsible for the remaining 20%, or $100 (Gordon and Gordon 2016a, 426–427).

82. a   Managed FFS reimbursement is similar to traditional FFS reimbursement except that managed care plans control costs primarily by managing their members' use of healthcare services (Gordon and Gordon 2016a, 429–430).

83. d   The case-mix index is 1.45 for the total case-mix index of the hospital. An individual MS-DRG case mix can be figured by multiplying the relative weight of each MS-DRG by the number of discharges within that MS-DRG. This provides the total weight for each MS-DRG. The sum of all total weights (15,192) divided by the sum of total patient discharges (10,471) equals the case-mix index (Horton 2016, 401).

84. d   Discounting applies to multiple surgical procedures furnished during the same operative session. The full rate will be paid to the surgical procedure with the highest rate and the additional procedures will be discounted 50% of their APC rate (Hazelwood and Venable 2016, 229).

85. b   Medicare Part B, also known as supplemental medical insurance, covers physicians and surgeons services and other Medicare-approved practitioners, ED and outpatient services, home health not covered under Part A, labs, x-rays, ASC services, physical and occupational therapies, and other services (Hazelwood and Venable 2016, 208).

86. d   Prior approval for a service or procedure is called precertification and allows coverage for a specific service (Casto and Forrestal 2015, 67, 101, 332–333).

87. d   Editing is not based on the clinical documentation of the discharge summary. Edits are predetermined based on coding conventions defined in the CPT codebooks, national and local policies and coding edits, analysis of standard medical and surgical practice, and review of current coding practices (Rinehart-Thompson 2016, 265).

88. a   Portions of the NCCI are incorporated into the outpatient code editor (OCE) against which all ambulatory claims are reviewed. The OCE also applies a set of logical rules to determine whether various combinations of codes are correct and appropriately represent services provided (Smith 2019, 58–59).

89. c   Outpatient claims editor does not exist. Do not confuse this terminology with outpatient code editor (OCE) (Smith 2019, 305).

90. b   Clean claims are essential for accurate and timely reimbursement (Casto and Forrestal 2015, 69).

91. a   Submitting paper claims subjects the claim to errors, whereas submitting electronic claims, using electronic health records, and auditing claims accuracy reduces the chance that the claim will contain inaccuracies or be incomplete (Casto and Forrestal 2015, 69, 71).

92. d   A procedure name is not a required element on a healthcare insurance claim (Casto and Forrestal 2015, 69–71).

93. a   VBID calculates both the benefit and the costs of clinical services (Casto and Forrestal 2015, 78).

94. a   The electronic format for institutional or facility claims is 837I for institutional claims, whereas 837P is for professional claims. The UB-04 and the 1500 forms are the paper billing forms for hospital (technical) and clinic (professional) claims, respectively (Casto and Forrestal 2015, 255).

95. a   Some Medicare beneficiaries choose to participate in the Medicare Advantage plan, which provides expanded coverage of many healthcare services via different plans including HMOs, PPOs, private for-service plans, and special need plans (Hazelwood and Venable 2016, 210).

96. c   Claims that automatically process through computer software either auto-pay, auto-suspend, or auto-deny (Casto and Forrestal 2015, 69).

97. b   Relative value units (RVUs) are assigned to each service to provide a value that correlates to payment (Casto and Forrestal 2015, 150–152).

98. d   A service must not be solely for the convenience of the insured, the insured's family, or the provider (Casto and Forrestal 2015, 65–66).

99. b   Coordination of benefits is necessary to determine which policy is primary and which is secondary so that there is no duplication of payments (Hazelwood and Venable 2016, 205).

100. b   A DRG is a predetermined amount of reimbursement for each Medicare inpatient (Hazelwood and Venable 2016, 223).

101. d   Medicare defines fraud as intentional deception or misrepresentation that results in an unauthorized benefit to an individual (Hazelwood and Venable 2012, 231).

102. c   The OIG investigates and prosecutes individuals who over-bill Medicare. It also develops an annual work plan that delineates the specific target areas that will be monitored in a given year (Hazelwood and Venable 2012, 230).

103. a   Physicians can prevent or minimize potentially abusive or fraudulent activities by developing a compliance plan (Hazelwood and Venable 2012, 231).

104. b   The case-mix index can be figured by multiplying the relative weight of each MS-DRG by the number of discharges within that MS-DRG (Hazelwood and Venable 2016, 232).

105. d   Eligibility standards for low income is a measure for Medicaid. Each state determines the standards according to federal guidelines (Hazelwood and Venable 2016, 210).

106. a   The Healthcare Common Procedural Coding System (HCPCS) identifies and groups the services within each APC group (Hazelwood and Venable 2016, 228–229).

107. c   The health information department along with the business office and cardiac department should be consulted to determine where the breakdown of the charges and assignment of the procedure code occurs. Often one department assumes another department is submitting the code or charge and without auditing and communicating with each other on a regular basis, error can occur for long periods of time with either a financial gain or loss to the facility (Casto and Forrestal 2015, 254, 264–265).

108. b   Medicare administrative contractors (MACs) are replacing the claims payment contractors known as FIs and carriers (Casto and Forrestal 2015, 255–256).

109. a   HCPCS codes that are assigned in the charge description master that flow directly to the claim and bypass facility coding staff is a process known as hard coding (Casto and Forrestal 2015, 253).

110. b   The person responsible for the bill is the *guarantor* (Casto and Forrestal 2015, 9, 324).

111. c   Clinical data document the patient's medical condition, diagnosis, and procedures performed as well as healthcare treatment provided (Brickner 2016, 88–90).

112. c   The operative report includes a description of the procedure performed (Brickner 2016, 95–96).

113. a   Results for lab tests will be included in a medical laboratory report (Brickner 2016, 94).

114. d   Results of an x-ray interpretation by a radiologist are reported in a radiography report (Brickner 2016, 94).

115. c   The American College of Surgeons developed the minimum standards for hospital health records in 1917 (Brickner 2016, 99).

116. b   Pathological examinations of tissue samples and tissues or organs removed during surgical procedures are reported in the pathology report (Brickner 2016, 94).

117. a   Physician orders are the instructions a physician gives to the other healthcare professionals. Admission and discharge orders should be found for every patient (Brickner 2016, 93).

118. c   This information is collected by the examination of a newborn and reported on the newborn record (Brickner 2016, 100).

119. c   An ECG is a report of an electrocardiogram of the heart (Brickner 2016, 94).

120. b   CMS established the Conditions of Participation, which are rules and regulations under which facilities are reviewed for medical necessity, compliance, and other decision making rules (Reynolds and Sharp 2016, 100).

121. d   After an initial assessment, documentation by other allied health professionals varies by specialty with appropriate content and frequency of recording (Brickner 2016, 90–93).

122. a   In 1974, the federal government adopted the UHDDS as the standard for collecting data for the Medicare and Medicaid programs. When the Prospective Payment Act was enacted in 1983, UHDDS definitions were incorporated into the rules and regulations for implementing diagnosis-related groups (DRGs). A key component was the incorporation of the definitions of principal diagnosis, principal procedure, and other significant procedures, into the DRG algorithms (Oachs and Watters 2016, 223).

123. b   CMS requires health records to be maintained for at least five years (42 CFR 482.24(b); Reynolds and Sharp 2016, 133)

124. a   Subjective information includes symptoms and actions reported by the patient and not observed or measured by the healthcare provider (Amatayakul 2016, 294).

125. b   Objective information may be measured or observed by the healthcare provider (Amatayakul 2016, 294).

126. d   The plan includes orders and the roadmap for patient care (Brickner 2016, 93).

127. c   Professional conclusions reached from evaluation of the subjective or objective information make up the assessment (Brickner 2016, 93–94).

128. a   HIM professionals analyze medical records for any missing reports, forms, or required signatures and deletions. This is a *quantitative analysis* of the medical record (Sayles 2016, 64).

129. c   Data currency and data timeliness refer to the requirement that healthcare data should be up-to-date and recorded at or near the time of the event or observation (Sayles 2016, 63–64).

130. b   Consistent data will be the same each time it is reported or collected (Sayles 2016, 63–64).

131. a   *Clinical data* document the patient's medical condition, diagnosis, and procedures performed as well as the healthcare treatment provided (Brickner 2016, 90).

132. a   Home health aides may assist the patient with activities of daily living such as bathing and housekeeping, which allows the patient to remain at home. Documentation of this type of intervention is also necessary (Kellogg 2016a, 38).

133. c   The emergency care record includes a pertinent history of the illness or injury and physical findings (Brickner 2016, 100).

134. d   The pathology report includes descriptions of the tissue from a gross or macroscopic level and representative cells at the microscopic level (Brickner 2016, 94).

135. d   The integrated health record is arranged so that the documentation from various sources is intermingled and follows strict chronological order (Brickner 2016, 82).

136. b   A complete medical history documents the patient's current complaints and symptoms and lists his or her past medical, personal, and family history (Brickner 2016, 90).

137. a   A physical examination report represents the attending physician's assessment of the patient's current health status (Brickner 2016, 91).

138. b   The consultation report documents the clinical opinion of a physician other than the primary or attending physician (Brickner 2016, 96).

139. c   Physician orders are the instructions the physician gives to the other healthcare professionals (Brickner 2016, 92–93).

140. a   Patient identity management relies on the Master Patient Index (Reynolds and Sharp 2016, 104).

141. a   In a joint effort of the Department of Health and Human Services (HHS), Office of Inspector General (OIG), Centers for Medicare and Medicaid Services (CMS), and Administration on Aging (AOA), Operation Restore Trust was released in 1995 to target fraud and abuse among healthcare providers (Casto and Forrestal 2015, 37).

142. d   Tracking length of stay is part of the hospital utilization review committee function (Casto and Forrestal 2015, 100–101).

143. c   Refiling claims after a denial is not possible because denied claims must be appealed and is not a factor in controlling fraud and abuse (Casto and Forrestal 2015, 36–38).

144. b   Benchmarking or peer comparison helps a manager to know how his or her team has performed compared to peers. This includes whether the case-mix index level puts the facility at risk (Casto and Forrestal 2015, 44).

145. c   Any inappropriate payment made to a healthcare organization for any reason is considered an improper or inappropriate payment. Mistakes are errors. Other types of inappropriate payments are inefficiencies, abuse, and fraud (Foltz et al. 2016, 448).

146. c   Within the Coding Compliance Plan, this is a strategy to combat fraud and abuse in coding (Foltz et al. 2016, 462).

147. c   *Encryption* is the process of transforming text into an unintelligible string of characters that can be transmitted via communications media with a high degree of security and then decrypted when it reaches a secure destination (Rinehart-Thompson 2016, 266).

148. d   *Data reliability* is a method of looking at data quality consistently. Reliability is frequently checked by having more than one person abstract data for the same case and compare the results for any discrepancies (Rinehart-Thompson 2016a, 260, 268).

149. c   HIPAA mandated incorporation of healthcare information standards into all electronic or computer-based health information systems (Rinehart-Thompson 2016b, 271).

150. a   HL7 developed the HL7 Electronic Health Record System (EHR-S) Functional Model. It also includes many standards for data exchange with patient information (Brinda 2016, 153).

151. a   Pay for performance and pay for quality are types of incentive to improve clinical performance (Gordon and Gordon 2016a, 439).

152. b   Computer viruses and other malware constitute a threat to data security (Rinehart-Thompson 2016c, 256–258).

153. b   Controlling access—facilities may authorize access to patient data in the facility's computer system to only those who need the access to do their job. This method of control serves the security of the data of patient records (Brinda 2016, 150–153).

154. b   An *audit trail* is a record of all transactions in the computer system, which is maintained and reviewed for instances of unauthorized access (Sayles 2016, 68).

155. c   The False Claims Act was passed during the Civil War. The law is the foundation upon which fraud and abuse efforts have been based (Foltz et al. 2016, 449).

156. c   Performance counseling usually begins with informal counseling or a verbal warning. No record is kept in the employee's file (Prater 2016, 574).

157. b   Establish a process, such as a hotline, to receive complaints and adopt procedures to protect the anonymity of complainants and to protect whistleblowers from retaliation (Prater 2016, 581–582).

158. d   All newly hired coding personnel should receive extensive training on the facility's and HIM department's compliance programs. Education of the medical staff on documentation is likewise important to the success of any compliance program (Prater 2016, 457, 556–558).

159. d   The OIG has issued compliance program guidance since 1998 (Foltz et al. 2016, 457).

160. c   *Upcoding* is the practice of assigning a diagnosis or procedure code specifically for the purpose of obtaining a higher level of payment (Foltz et al. 2016, 458–462).

161. d   A *compliance officer* designs, implements, and maintains a compliance program that assures conformity to all types of regulatory and voluntary accreditation requirements governing the provision of healthcare products and services (Foltz et al. 2016, 457).

162. b   *Concurrent review* occurs on a continuing basis during a patient's stay (Foltz et al. 2016, 459–461).

163. a   Health Information Portability and Accountability Act of 1996 (Rinehart-Thompson 2016, 214).

164. b   The mission of the OIG is to protect the integrity of the DHHS defined by the strategic plan (Palkie 2016, 292).

165. d   A joint effort of the HHS and DOJ, the mission of this program is to prevent waste, fraud and abuse, reduce health care costs, improve quality of care for Medicare and Medicaid patients, and provide best practice information (Foltz et al. 2016, 451).

166. d Disclosures for which accounting is not required involve nine exceptions including those in the question (Rinehart-Thompson 2016, 214).

167. b Notices of privacy must be posted in a prominent place where it is reasonable to expect that patients will read them (Gordon and Gordon 2016b, 609–610).

168. a An *incidental disclosure* occurs as part of a permitted use of disclosure (Gordon and Gordon 2016b, 214, 615–616).

169. b Data quality includes the following characteristics: accuracy, accessibility, comprehensiveness, consistency, currency, definition, granularity, precision, relevancy, and timeliness (Rinehart-Thompson 2016, 260, 268).

170. b *Data security* is the means of ensuring that data are kept safe from corruption and that access to data is suitably controlled (Rinehart-Thompson 2016, 256–258).

171. c The type of tool used to aid in the coding process is called an encoder (Sayles 2016, 75).

172. d A *portal* is a special application to provide secure remote access to specific applications (Amatayakul 2016, 287).

173. b There are several different types of computer-assisted coding (CAC), including software to aid the physicians (Sayles 2016, 75).

174. b *Natural-language processing* (NLP) is an artificial intelligence software that reads digital text from online documents and suggests codes to match the documentation (Sayles 2016, 69).

175. d The ONC developed the vision and mission with direction from the federal government's Federal Health IT Strategic Plan 2015–2020 (Amatayakul 2016, 285).

176. d The primary EHR applications include clinical documentation or patient care charting, computerized provider order entry, electronic medical administration records, and clinical decision support (Sayles 2016, 53; Amatayakul 2016, 285).

177. a *Data definition* means that the data and information documented in the health record are defined; users of the data must understand what the data mean and represent (Sayles 2016, 52).

178. b Some encoders are built using expert system techniques such as rule-based systems, and other encoding software is more simplistic, merely automating a look-up function similar to the manual index in ICD or other coding classifications (Brinda 2016, 162).

179. a Good encoding software should include edit checks to ensure data quality (Brinda 2016, 162).

180. a Communications and network technologies—used by providers to enter orders for medications, lab tests, and other services—are the computerized provider order entry system (CPOE) (Amatayakul 2016, 287).

181. b One potential area for poor data quality surrounds the need for making data entry easier. These include "copy and paste," "macros," standard orders, and other techniques that "reuse" data. These techniques can make data entry faster, but care must be taken to ensure appropriate modification to the specific patient (Rinehart-Thompson 2016b, 243–245).

182. b For hospitals that do not have all EHR components, the result is a hybrid record that is part electronic and part paper. Some hospitals overcome hybrid record issues by scanning all paper documents into an EDMS, thereby making everything available online (Sayles and Gordon 2016, 53).

183. b Electronic signature authentication systems require the author to sign onto the system using a user ID and password, review the document to be signed, and indicate approval (Sayles 2016, 89).

184. d In both the MS-DRG and APC groupings, coders enter the codes that have been selected in a computer program called a grouper. The grouper then assigns the patient's case to the correct group based on the ICD-10-CM or CPT/HCPCS codes (Sayles 2016, 75).

185. b *Confidentiality* is a legal ethical concept that establishes the healthcare provider's responsibility for protecting health records and other personal and private information from unauthorized use or disclosure (Brodnik et al. 2012, 5–6).

186. d The UHCDA suggests that decision-making priority for an individual's next-of-kin be as follows: Spouse, adult child, parent, adult sibling, or if no one is available who is so related to the individual, authority may be granted to "an adult who exhibited special care and concern for the individual" (Brodnik et al. 2012, 332–333).

187. b A *subpoena* is a direct command that requires an individual or a representative of an organization to appear in court or to present an object to the court (Fahrenholz and Russo 2013, 94).

188. a The law permits a presumption of consent during emergency situations, regardless of whether the patient is an adult or a minor (Brodnik et al. 2012, 352).

189. b The Privacy Rule introduced the standard of minimum necessary to limit the amount of PHI used, disclosed, and requested. This means that healthcare providers and other covered entities must limit uses, disclosures, and requests to only the amount needed to accomplish the intended purpose (Rinehart-Thompson 2016b, 218).

190. a The HIPAA Privacy Rule provides patients with rights that allow them to have some control over their health information: right of access, right to request amendment of PHI, right to accounting of disclosures, right to request restrictions of PHI, right to request confidential communications, and right to complain of Privacy Rule violations (Rinehart-Thompson 2016b, 218).

191. c *Expressed consent* can be spoken or written (Rinehart-Thompson 2016c, 200; Rinehart-Thompson 2016b, 231).

192. a It is generally agreed that social security numbers (SSNs) should not be used as patient identifiers (Sayles 2016, 59).

193. b Deidentified information is information that does not identify an individual; essentially it is information from which personal characteristics have been stripped (Rinehart-Thompson 2016b, 222).

194. c The notice of privacy includes a statement that the covered entity reserves the right to change the terms of its notice and to make the new notice provisions effective for all PHI that it maintains (Rinehart-Thompson 2016b, 230).

195. d   Although e-Discovery is the same pretrial process as discovery, the electronic health record has promoted this concept (Rinehart-Thompson 2016b, 215).

196. c   *Subpoena duces tecum* is a written document directing individuals or organizations to furnish relevant documents and records (Rinehart-Thompson 2016b, 215).

197. c   A covered entity must act on an individual's request for review of PHI no later than 30 days after the request is made (Rinehart-Thompson 2016b, 220).

198. a   The standard of minimum necessary means that healthcare providers and other covered entities must limit uses, disclosures, and requests to only the amount needed to accomplish the intended purpose (Rinehart-Thompson 2016b, 220).

199. b   Under the Privacy Rule, healthcare providers are not required to obtain patient consent to use or disclose personally identifiable information for treatment, payment, or healthcare operations (Rinehart-Thompson 2016b, 218).

200. b   The agreement between the covered entity and business associate should, at termination of the contract, require the business associate to return or destroy all PHI received from the covered entity that it still maintains and prohibit the associate from retaining it (Rinehart-Thompson 2016b, 220).

CCA Practice Exam 1

1. d   Index Fracture, traumatic, femur, capital epiphyseal. Seventh character is required for further classification of an episode of care and the healing status (Schraffenberger 2018, 574–578).

2. d   Index either Neonatal, tooth, teeth K00.6, or Eruption, teeth/tooth (Schraffenberger 2018, 365–367).

3. a   CPT code 21012 describes excision of a subcutaneous soft tissue tumor of the face or scalp greater than 2 cm and is appropriately coded when the tumor is removed from the subcutaneous tissue rather than subgaleal or intramuscular. Simple and intermediate closure of the wound is included in the procedure for the excision in the musculoskeletal section of CPT (AMA 2018, 116).

4. c   Code 19125 describes an excision of a lesion that was identified by preoperative placement of a radiological marker (AMA 2018, 103–104).

5. a   Four-digit codes are available to classify Alzheimer's disease with early onset G30.0 (Schraffenberger 2018, 225).

6. d   ICD-10-PCS classifies cardiac pacemakers as Devices, character 6. Root operations of Insertion, removal, and revision always involve a device, such as a pacemaker. In coding initial insertion of a dual chamber permanent pacemaker, three codes are required—one for the pacemaker (0JH606Z) and one for each lead (02H63JZ, 02HK3JZ) (Schraffenberger 2018, 51, 68–70).

7. a   When a pacemaker is replaced with another pacemaker, both the removal of the old device and the insertion of the new pacemaker are coded (0JPT0PZ, 0JH606Z). Per ICD-10-PCS Reference Manual, 2.55, "A procedure to remove a device is coded to Removal if it is not an integral part of another root operation." It is not coded to the root operation Change because this involved cutting the skin. Change is only used for External approaches (CMS 2018).

8. b ICD-10-CM classifies both Mobitz type I and type II to I44.1 (Schraffenberger 2018, 314).

9. a Index Checking (of), cardiac pacemaker, pulse generator, Z45.010. The pacemaker check is the root operation Measurement. Index: Measurement, Cardiac, Pacemaker 4B02XSZ (Schraffenberger 2018, 57–60, 654–655).

10. c Coding Guideline I.C.9.a.2 states to assign codes from category I12, when both hypertension and a condition classifiable to category N18, Chronic kidney disease (CKD), are present (CMS 2018a).

11. c Index Bypass, Artery, Coronary, One artery. One artery is selected since there two different Qualifiers (Character 7). One Qualifier is "8 Internal Mammary, Right," and the other is "9 Internal Mammary, Left." Internal mammary-coronary artery bypass is accomplished by loosening the internal mammary artery from its normal position and using the internal mammary artery to bring blood from the subclavian artery to the occluded coronary artery. Codes are selected based on whether one or both internal mammary arteries are used (Schraffenberger 2018, 68–70).

12. c The Judkins technique provides x-ray imaging of the coronary arteries by introducing one catheter into the femoral artery with maneuvering up into the left coronary artery orifice, followed by a second catheter guided up into the right coronary artery, and subsequent injection of a contrast material (Schraffenberger 2018, 321–323).

13. a Z51.81, Encounter for, Therapeutic drug monitoring, is the correct code to use when a patient visit is for the sole purpose of undergoing a laboratory test to measure the drug level in the patient's blood or urine or to measure a specific function to assess the effectiveness of the drug. Z51.81 may be used alone if the monitoring is for a drug that the patient is on for only a brief period, not long term. However, there is a "code also" note under this code to remind the coder to code for any associated long-term current drug use with codes from category Z79 (Schraffenberger 2018, 682).

14. b Code 25810 is assigned to report arthrodesis of wrist, complete, with iliac autograft or other autograft (including obtaining graft) (AMA 2018, 152).

15. c Code 43761 describes the repositioning of the nasograstric tube. If imaging guidance is performed, assign 76000 (AMA 2018, 318).

16. c An incomplete abortion is one in which some, but not all, of the products of conception are expulsed from the uterus. If the placenta or secundines remain, the abortion is considered incomplete (Schraffenberger 2018, 493).

17. b Index Abortion, threatened (spontaneous) O20.0. Hemorrhage is included in the code per the Includes notes under O20.0. Category Z3A, Weeks of gestation, is assigned as an additional code for all pregnancy and childbirth codes per the "use additional code" note at the beginning of Chapter 15 (Schraffenberger 2018, 496–497, 488).

18. a Index Delivery, complicated, by, dilation, cervix incomplete, poor, or slow (O62.0). Outcome of delivery, single, liveborn (Z37.0) is assigned as an additional code. Code Z3A.40, 40 weeks of gestation is assigned as an additional code per the "use additional code" note at the beginning of Chapter 15. Cesarean section, low uterine segment is found in section 1 "Obstetrics" of the Medical and Surgical Related section of the ICD-10-PCS book. The body system is 0, Pregnancy and the body part is products of conception. The qualifier specifies the type of Cesarean (1 low, in this case) (Schraffenberger 2018, 477, 482–486, 678).

19. b   Index Rash, diaper, L22 (Schraffenberger 2018, 395–396).

20. c   Coding Guideline I.C.12.a.5 notes that pressure ulcers present on admission but healed at the time of discharge are assigned the code for site and stage at time of admission.

21. b   Index, Osteoarthritis, primary, hip, bilateral (Schraffenberger 2018, 425–426).

22. a   Index Chondromalacia, patella M22.4– (Schraffenberger 2018, 427).

23. a.   Excision of benign lesions of skin includes margins and simple closure. Code selection is determined by measuring the greatest clinical diameter of the lesion plus the margin (AMA 2018, 83).

24. a   Index tetralogy of Fallot Q21.3. Since this is newborn transfer, Z code is not assigned (CMS CG 16a2).

25. b   Index Anemia, aplastic, due to, drugs, D61.1. A coder should always assign the most specific type of anemia. Anemia due to chemotherapy is often aplastic. There is a "use additional code for adverse effect" note at D61.1 to assign an additional code to identify the drug causing the anemia. Utilize the Table of Drugs and Chemicals to locate the term Antineoplastic NEC. Then follow the row across to the Adverse effect column to locate the code. A seventh character of "A" is used to indicate "initial encounter" (Schraffenberger 2018, 140).

26. c   Index Examination, well baby, Z00.129 for the routine well-child examination. Index, Premature, infant—See Preterm, newborn, unspecified weeks of gestation. P07.30 is assigned as an additional code per Guideline I.C.16.e (Schraffenberger 2018, 515, 646–647).

27. d   Index Dysfunction, ventricular I51.9 (Schraffenberger 2018, 290–291).

28. c   Certain signs and symptoms of breast disease are included in category N64 Other disorders of breast, which are in Chapter 14 Diseases of the genitourinary system (Schraffenberger 2018, 456).

29. c   Index Bunionectomy, see Excision, Lower Bones table 0QB. Locate table 0QB. Then select N Metatarsal, right for the Body Part (character 4), and select 0 Open for the Approach (character 5), and select Z No Device for Device (character 6), and select Z No Qualifier for the Qualifier (character 7) (CMS 2018, 955; Schraffenberger 2018, 434–440).

30. a   Per Coding Guideline I.C.12.a.6, if a patient is admitted with a pressure ulcer at one stage and it progresses to a higher stage, two separate codes should be assigned: one code for the site and stage on admission and a second code for the same site at the highest stage (CMS 2018a).

31. d   Index Cholecystectomy, see Resection, Gallbladder, table 0FT4 because the whole gallbladder was removed. The laparoscopy is the approach and is not coded separately per 2014 ICD-10-PCS Official Guidelines for Coding and Reporting, Guideline B3.11a (page 8) "Inspection of a body part performed in order to achieve the objective of a procedure is not coded separately." To build the code, locate table 0FT and body part 4 Gallbladder, then 4 Percutaneous Endoscopic for the approach, then Z No device for device, and Z No qualifier for the qualifier (Schraffenberger 2018, 76–77).

32. c Index Excision, Bladder, table 0TBB since a portion of the bladder was removed. The cystoscopy is the approach—via natural or artificial opening, endoscopic. Final code assignment is 0TBB8ZX. The qualifier of "X Diagnostic" is used for biopsies (Schraffenberger 2018, 60–61, 384).

33. b An *encoder* is a computer software program designed to assist coders in assigning appropriate clinical codes and helps ensure accurate reporting of diagnoses and procedures (Sayles 2016, 75).

34. b The RBRVS system is the federal government's payment system for physicians. It is a system of classifying health services based on the cost of furnishing physicians' services in different settings, the skill and training levels required to perform the services, and the time and risk involved (Casto and Forrestal 2015, 6, 10, 149).

35. c Tricare is the healthcare program for active duty members of the military and other qualified family members (Hazelwood and Venable 2016, 213).

36. b *CPT Assistant* provides additional CPT coding guidance on how to assign a CPT code by providing intent on the use of the code and explanation of parenthetical instructions. The American Medical Association publishes the guidance monthly (AMA 2018, xvii).

37. b *Unbundling* occurs when a panel code exists, and the individual tests are reported rather than the panel code (Smith 2019, 67).

38. a Reporting additional test codes that overlap codes in a panel allows the coder to assign all appropriate codes for services provided. It is inappropriate to assign additional panel codes when all codes in the panel are not performed. Reporting individual lab codes is appropriate when all codes in a panel have not been provided (Smith 2019, 204).

39. a Clustering is coding or charging one or two middle levels of service codes exclusively (Hazelwood and Venable 2014, 231–232).

40. b The front end of the RCM process includes scheduling and registration, insurance verification, preauthorization, financial counseling and pre-encounter services. Claims appeals are a back end process (Malmgren and Solberg 2016, 245).

41. c AHA's *Coding Clinic for ICD-10-CM/PCS* is a quarterly publication of the Central Office on ICD-10-CM/PCS, which allows coders to submit a request for coding advice through the coding publication. AHA Coding Clinic is the only official publication for ICD-10-CM/PCS coding guidelines and advice provided by the four Cooperating Parties (Hazelwood and Venable 2014, 12).

42. b CMS developed MUEs to prevent providers from billing units in excess and receiving inappropriate payments. This new editing was the result of the outpatient prospective payment system that pays providers passed on the HCPCS/CPT code and units. Payment is directly related to units for specified HCPCS/CPT codes assigned to an ambulatory payment classification (CMS 2017c, I-5–I-6).

43. c The documentation of the charges and itemized bill is not the responsibility of the physician (Smith 2019, 9–10).

44. d   The identity of the patient's nearest relative and an emergency contact number are not relative to securing payment from the insurer. The encounter should include the date of the encounter and the identity of the observer (Smith 2019, 9–10).

45. b   The hospital will receive the same reimbursement regardless of the length of stay (Casto and Forrestal 2015, 116, 121).

46. a   Higher relative weights link to higher payment rates (Casto and Forrestal 2015, 115).

47. c   Home health resource groups (HHRGs) represent the classification system established for the prospective reimbursement of covered home care services to Medicare beneficiaries during a 60-day episode of care (Gordon and Gordon 2016a, 442).

48. c   The resource-based relative value scale (RBRVS) system was implemented by CMS in 1992 for physicians' services such as office visits covered under Medicare Part B. The system reimburses physicians according to a fee schedule based on predetermined values assigned to specific services (Gordon and Gordon 2016a, 441).

49. c   Major diagnostic categories (MDCs), of which there are 25. The principal diagnosis determines the MDC assignment (Hazelwood and Venable 2016, 223).

50. a   Children's hospitals are excluded from PPS because the PPS diagnosis-related groups do not accurately account for the resource costs for the types of patients treated (Gordon and Gordon 2016a, 440).

51. c   CMS identified *hospital-acquired conditions* (not present on admission) as "reasonably preventable," and hospitals do not receive additional payment for cases in which these conditions are not present on admission (Horton 2016, 399).

52. c   Gram-negative pneumonia is not on CMS's list of diagnoses that are considered to be hospital-acquired conditions (HACs). HACs (not present on admission) are considered to be "reasonably preventable," and hospitals do not receive additional payment for cases in which one of the conditions was not present on admission (Hazelwood and Venable 2016, 226).

53. a   Stage I and II pressure ulcers are not considered hospital-acquired conditions but stage III and IV are (Hazelwood and Venable 2016, 226).

54. b   The electronic claim form (screen 837I) replaced the UB-04 (CMS 1450) paper billing form (Smith 2019, 11–15).

55. b   An EOB is a statement sent by a third-party payer to the patient to explain the services provided (Hazelwood and Venable 2016, 235).

56. c   Uniform Ambulatory Care Data Set (Fahrenholz and Russo 2013, 295–298).

57. c   *Vocabulary standards* establish common definitions for medical terms to encourage consistent descriptions of an individual's condition in the health record (Giannangelo 2016, 114).

58. a   The *consultation report* documents the clinical opinion of a physician other than the primary or attending physician. The report is based on the consulting physician's examination of the patient and a review of his or her health record (Brickner 2016, 90, 96).

59. a   The *discharge summary* provides an overview of the entire medical encounter to ensure the continuity of future care by providing information to the patient's attending physician, referring physician, and any consulting physicians, to provide information to support the activities of the medical staff review committee and to provide concise information that can be used to answer information requests from authorized individuals or entities (Brickner 2016, 97).

60. b   Under HIPAA, at the time of admission or prior to treatment, patients must be informed about the use of individually identifiable health information. This form is signed by the patient (Reynolds and Sharp 2016, 105).

61. c   The nature and duration of the symptoms that caused the patient to seek medical attention as stated in the patient's own words (Fahrenholz and Russo 2013, 203).

62. a   *Clinical information* is data related to the patient's diagnosis or treatment in a healthcare facility (Fahrenholz and Russo 2013, 77, 197–198).

63. d   Financial data include details about the patient's occupation, employer, and insurance coverage (Fahrenholz and Russo 2013, 76–77, 189–190).

64. c   The *Subjective, Objective, Assessment, Plan (SOAP)* notes are part of the problem-oriented health record approach most commonly used by physicians and other healthcare professionals. SOAP notes are intended to improve the quality and continuity of client services by enhancing communication among healthcare professionals (Fahrenholz and Russo 2013, 304–305).

65. c   Focus charting, or charting by exception, is a method of documenting only abnormal or unusual findings or deviations from the patient's plan of care (Reynolds and Sharp 2016, 112).

66. a   The transfer or referral form provides document communication between caregivers in multiple healthcare settings. It is important that a patient's treatment plan be consistent as the patient moves through the healthcare delivery system (Fahrenholz and Russo 2013, 225).

67. c   According to the Joint Commission, except in emergency situations, every surgical patient's chart must include a report of a complete history and physical conducted no more than seven days before the surgery is to be performed (Fahrenholz and Russo 2013, 238).

68. a   According to Medicare Conditions of Participation, the physical examination must be completed within 24 hours of admission (Fahrenholz and Russo 2013, 200).

69. b   An incomplete record not rectified within a specific number of days as indicated in the medical staff rules and regulations is considered to be delinquent (Sayles 2016, 65).

70. b   A complete medical history documents the patient's current complaints and symptoms and lists the patient's past medical, social, and family history (Brickner 2016, 90).

71. b   The benefit of concurrent review is that content or authentication issues can be identified at the time of patient care and rectified in a timely manner (Sayles 2016 64, 438).

72. c   The HIM manager may compare organizational data with external data from peer groups to determine best practices (Carter and Palmer 2016, 508).

73. d   Surveyors review the documentation of patient care services to determine whether the standards for care are being met (Brickner 2016, 82–87).

74. c   Participating organizations must follow the Medicare Conditions of Participation to receive federal funds from the Medicare program for services rendered (Brickner 2016, 84, 102).

75. b   Every healthcare facility should have a compliance program, a set of internal policies and procedures that are put into place to comply with federal and state laws (Brickner 2016, 457).

76. b   The pathology report describes specimens examined by the pathologist (Amatayakul 2016, 287).

77. d   It is not appropriate for the coder to assume the removal was done by either snare or hot biopsy forceps. The ablation code is only assigned when a lesion is completely destroyed and no specimen is retrieved. The coding professional must query the physician to assign the appropriate code (AHIMA 2016, 454).

78. d   The RAC demonstration uncovered $1.03 billion of improper payments, of which 96 percent were overpayments and 4 percent were underpayments (Casto and Forrestal 2015, 38, 40–42).

79. c   Seven elements are required as part of the basic elements of a corporate compliance program. A medical staff appointee is not one of these required elements (Foltz et al. 2016, 457).

80. d   Quality improvement (QI) programs have been in place in hospitals for years and have been required by the Medicare or Medicaid programs and accreditation standards. QI programs have covered medical staff as well as nursing and other departments or processes (O'Dell 2016, 657).

81. b   Hospitals are encouraged but not required to follow the same work plan as the OIG. Hospitals should review the plan carefully and plan their compliance program around the target areas (Foltz et al. 2016, 457).

82. a   The coder is not following Standard 6 of AHIMA Standards of Ethical Coding, which states that all healthcare data elements required for external reporting purposes, including quality and patient safety measurements, are to be reported (Gordon and Gordon 2016b, 616–617).

83. c   The OIG believes that compliance programs will benefit by identifying and preventing criminal and unethical conduct, in addition to the other benefits listed (Palkie 2016, 297, 304).

84. c   *Medical identity theft* occurs when someone uses a person's name and sometimes other parts of their identity without the victim's knowledge or consent to obtain medical services or goods (Palkie 2016, 295).

85. b   With an automated tracking system, it is easy to track how many records are charged out of the system, their location, and whether they have been returned on the due dates indicated (Amatayakul 2016, 304–307).

86. a   Audit trails can provide tracking information such as who accessed which records and for what purpose (Sandefer 2016, 366).

87. a   Role-based access control (RBAC) is a control system in which access decisions are based on the roles of individual users as part of an organization (Brodnik et al. 2012, 304).

88. a   Encoders come in two distinct categories: logic-based and automated codebook formats. A *logic-based encoder* prompts the user through a variety of questions and choices based on the clinical terminology entered. The coder selects the most accurate code for a service or condition (and any possible complications or comorbidities). An *automated codebook* provides screen views that resemble the actual format of the coding system (Sayles 2016, 75).

89. d   EDI allows the transfer (incoming and outgoing) of information directly from one computer to another by using standard formats (Sayles 2016, 68–76).

90. c   New systems are continuously updated to meet the needs of the facilities. Various states include implementation, meaningful use, adoption and optimization (Amatayakul 2016, 288).

91. a   *Clinical decision support* includes providing documentation of clinical findings and procedures, active reminders about medication administration, suggestions for prescribing less expensive but equally effective drugs, protocols for certain health maintenance procedures, alerts that a duplicate lab test is being ordered, and countless other decision-making aids for all stakeholders in the care process (Sayles 2016, 76).

92. b   A consolidated federated model has independent vaults or databases managed by the health information organization (HIO) so that data are centrally managed but both logically and physically separated (Amatayakul 2016, 306–307).

93. c   The designated record set includes health records that are used to make decisions about the individual (Sayles 2016, 53–55).

94. a   The covered entity must provide access to the personal health information in the form or format requested when it is readily producible in such form or format. When it is not readily producible in the form or format requested, it must be produced in a readable hard-copy form or such other form or format agreed upon by the covered entity and the individual (Gordon and Gordon 2016b, 615–616).

95. c   A healthcare organization involved in litigation will involve fact-finding. Discovery is a pre-trial stage that includes the deposition of oral testimonies of parties to the lawsuit (Rinehart-Thompson 2016b, 214).

96. c   Because federal regulations such as HIPAA and state laws govern the release of health record information, HIM department personnel must know what information needs to be included on the authorization for it to be considered valid (Gordon and Gordon 2016b, 615–616).

97. b   It is suggested that covered entities use PHI with certain specified direct identifiers removed as a guideline for disclosing only minimum necessary information while providing the amount needed to accomplish the intended purpose (Gordon and Gordon 2016b, 615–616).

98. b   *Privacy* is the right of an individual to be left alone. It includes freedom from observation or intrusion into one's private affairs and the right to maintain control over certain personal and health information (Rinehart-Thompson 2016b, 214; Gordon and Gordon 2016b, 610).

99. d   Data integrity services ensure the data are not altered as they are stored or transmitted electronically (Brinda 2016, 152; Rinehart-Thompson 2016a, 254).

100. d   Security measures not only provide for confidentiality, but data integrity and data availability— the CIA of security (Rinehart-Thompson 2016a, 258).

CCA Practice Exam 2

1. c   The residual condition or nature of the sequela is sequenced first, followed by the cause of the sequela (Hazelwood and Venable 2014, 5, 181). The seventh character "S" is added to the laceration code to identify the sequela.

2. c   Index Dysphagia, following, cerebral infarction I69.391. Add R13.10 as an additional code per "use additional code to identify the type of dysphagia, if known (R13.1-)" note under I69.391. Multiple codes may be needed for sequelae...in order to fully describe a condition. In the Tabular List, the instruction of "Use additional code" note indicates it is necessary to assign a secondary code to fully describe a condition or disease process (Hazelwood and Venable 2014, 4, 82).

3. b   Traumatic amputation classified in chapter 19. Index Traumatic amputation, finger (complete metacarpophalangeal) S68.11-. 7th character "A" initial encounter (Schraffenberger, 2018, 590).

4. d   Index Elevated, elevation, prostate specific antigen (PSA), R97.20 (Hazelwood and Venable 2014, 173).

5. b   Near-syncope and nausea are both symptoms and therefore not integral to the other. Both conditions should be coded (Hazelwood and Venable 2014, 172–173).

6. d   An oral glucose tolerance test helps determine whether a patient has prediabetes or diabetes. Index Elevated, elevation, glucose tolerance (oral) R73.02, which when verified in the Tabular, is a complete code. The Tabular should always be referenced to verify the code (Hazelwood and Venable 2014, 46).

7. c   Pneumonia, unspecified, is assigned J18.9 in the Alphabetic Index. The persistent cough is a symptom of the pneumonia and should not be coded separately (Hazelwood and Venable 2014, 86–88).

8. a   Code signs and symptoms when a condition is *ruled out,* which means the condition has been proven not to exist. The code for seizures (R56.9) is assigned when a more specific diagnosis cannot be made even after all the facts bearing on the case have been investigated (Hazelwood and Venable 2014, 60, 173–174).

9. c   Urinary incontinence is a loss of urine without warning and may be associated with many conditions. ICD-10-CM classifies stress incontinence to N39.3 for both male and female types. Index Incontinence, stress (female) (male), N39.3. Subcategory N39.4, Other specified urinary incontinence, provides additional specificity that is not documented in this case.

    Code N39.46 Mixed incontinence is not correct because it includes urge incontinence in addition to stress. The patient only had stress incontinence. Codes R32 Unspecified urinary incontinence is not correct due to Excludes 1 note which excludes N39.3, Code N39.498 Other specified urinary incontinence is not correct because the type (stress) has a specific code (Hazelwood and Venable 2014, 130).

10. c   Category Z16, Resistance to Antimicrobial Drugs, is used as additional code. Assign sepsis for principal as "code first the infection." (Schraffenberger, 2018, 671).

11. **a**   Parentheses enclose supplementary words or explanatory information that may or may not be present in the statement of a diagnosis or procedure. They do not affect the code number assigned in the case. Bronchiectasis (fusiform) (postinfectious) (recurrent) is an example of a diagnosis statement with nonessential modifiers noted with parentheses (Schraffenberger 2018, 23).

12. **b**   Index Infarction, myocardium, myocardial, ST elevation (STEMI), anterior (anteroapical) (anterolateral) (anteroseptal) (Q wave) (wall) I21.09. There is no mention of a prior infarction within the last 28 days, so category I21 is appropriate. See Includes note under I21 (Schraffenberger 2018, 290–291, 295, 305–307).

13. **d**   Only confirmed cases of HIV infection or illness are reported, using code B20, Human immunodeficiency virus (HIV) disease per ICD-10-CM Official Guidelines for Coding and Reporting, Guideline I.C.1.a.1 (CMS 2018a).

      Patients with an HIV-related illness should be coded to category B20, which includes AIDS, AIDS-like syndrome, AIDS-related complex, and symptomatic HIV infection. When a patient is seen for an HIV-related condition, B20 Human immunodeficiency virus is the first listed diagnosis code. Any HIV-related conditions should be listed as additional diagnosis codes (Hazelwood and Venable 2014, 24).

14. **b**   The connecting term "due to" connects the organism *E. coli* to the urinary tract infection. The instructional note "Use additional code" (B95–B97) is found in the Tabular List of ICD-10-CM under Code N39.0. This notation indicates that use of an additional code may provide a more complete picture of the diagnosis or procedure. The additional code should always be assigned if the health record provides supportive documentation. Infection, urinary (tract) Tabular List—use additional code to identify organism. Infection, *Escherichia coli*. Index: Infection, Escherichia (E.) coli NEC, as cause of disease classified elsewhere B96.20 (Schraffenberger 2018, 20, 28–30, 126).

15. **a**   Per Coding Guideline I.C.13.c, the 7th character A is used as long as the patient is receiving active treatment for the fracture. While the patient may be seen by a new or different provider over the course of treatment for the pathological fracture, assignment of the 7th character is based on whether the patient is undergoing active treatment and not whether the provider is seeing the patient for the first time (CMS 2018a).

16. **c**   The terms *metastatic to* and *direct extension to* are used for classifying secondary malignant neoplasms in ICD-10-CM. For example, cancer described as "metastatic to a specific site" is interpreted as a secondary neoplasm of that site. The colon (C18.9) is the primary site, and the left lung (C78.02) is the secondary site (Hazelwood and Venable 2014, 30, 32–34).

17. **a**   Index: Sepsis, Staphylococcus, staphylococcal, aureus (methicillin susceptible) (MSSA) A41.01. Sepsis is the systemic infection. Because the organism is indicated in the sepsis code, B95.61 is redundant and should not be coded (Schraffenberger 2018, 111, 113–118).

18. **c**   ICD-10-CM classifies inadequately controlled, out of control, and poorly controlled diabetes mellitus as "*code* to diabetes, by type, with hyperglycemia." In this case, diabetes, diabetic, type 2, with, hyperglycemia. Malnutrition, mild, not stated as related to diabetes Index: Malnutrition, degree, mild E44.1 (Schraffenberger 2018, 180–182, 185–187, 189–190).

19. **d**   D70.9, Fever, neutropenic. Instructional note under D70 states to use additional code for any associated fever (R50.81) (Schraffenberger 2018, 162, 171).

20. a Both counseling and coordination of care are contributing factors in the selection of an E/M level of service. When counseling and coordination of care constitute more than 50 percent of the face-to-face time, time may be considered the key or controlling factor (Smith 2019, 250).

21. b New technology is addressed by the Category III codes (Smith 2019, 4).

22. b Because a separate procedure is considered a part of, and integral to, another, larger procedure, it is not coded when performed as part of the more extensive procedure. See Surgery Guidelines. It may, however, be coded when it is not performed as part of another, larger service; therefore, answer "c" is not correct (AHIMA 2016, 437).

23. b The AMA developed and maintains CPT. CMS developed and maintains HCPCS Level II codes (AHIMA 2016, 438).

24. c Any physician may use the codes in any section of CPT (AHIMA 2016, 438).

25. d See instructional notes preceding code 99217. In order to report these codes, the admission order must designate observation status. Whether the patient meets admission criteria or is admitted following surgery does not affect the observation code selection. If the patient is admitted and discharged on the same date, codes 99234–99236 are appropriate (AMA 2017, 14).

26. b Documentation of history of use of drugs, alcohol, and tobacco is considered part of the social history. The review of systems is a part of the history of present illness. See E/M Services Guidelines, instructions for selecting a level of E/M service, in the CPT manual (AMA 2018, 4–10).

27. c Tissue transplanted from one individual to another of the same species but different genotype is called an *allograft* or *allogeneic graft* (Kuehn and Jorwic 2019, 15).

28. b See definitions preceding code 17311 (Mohs micrographic technique) in CPT Professional Edition (AMA 2017, 98).

29. a The "with manipulation" code is used because the fracture was manipulated, even if the manipulation did not result in clinical anatomic alignment. See Musculoskeletal Guidelines, Definitions (AHIMA 2016, 446).

30. d Newborn care services are used to report the services provided to newborns in several different settings. For the newborn admitted and discharged on the same day, E/M code assignment per day is 99463 (AMA 2017, 42).

31. a If the tip of the catheter is manipulated, it is a selective catheterization. In the case of a nonselective catheterization, the tip of the catheter remains in either the aorta or the artery that was originally entered (AHIMA 2016, 451).

32. a See instructional note preceding code 36000 for Vascular Injection Procedures (AMA, 2018, 258).

33. b Diagnosis codes are often the primary reason for a service to be considered covered or denied by the insurance company. Local and national policies include diagnosis codes that are used in software edits to automatically deny or approve processed claims. Denied services can be appealed, and the record can be submitted to support medical necessity if the service fails the automated review (Schraffenberger 2018, 707–709).

34. b   The NUBC was established with the goal of developing an acceptable, uniform bill that would consolidate the numerous billing forms hospitals were required to use (Schraffenberger 2018, 89).

35. c   The Uniform Hospital Discharge Data Set was promulgated by the US Department of Health, Education, and Welfare in 1974 as a minimum, common core of data on individual acute-care, short-term hospital discharges in Medicare and Medicaid programs. It sought to improve the uniformity and comparability of hospital discharge data. In 1985, the data were expanded to include all non-outpatient settings (Schraffenberger 2018, 89–91).

36. a   For fiscal year 2008, Medicare adopted a severity-adjusted diagnosis-related groups system called Medicare Severity-DRGs (MS-DRGs). This was the most drastic revision to the DRG system in 24 years. The goal of the new MS-DRG system was to significantly improve Medicare's ability to recognize severity of illness in its inpatient hospital payments. The new system is projected to increase payments to hospitals for services provided to the sicker patients and decrease payments for treating less severely ill patients (Schraffenberger 2018, 702).

37. a   For any given patient in a MS-DRG, the hospital knows, in advance, the amount of reimbursement it will receive from Medicare. It is the responsibility of the hospital to ensure that its resource use is in line with the payment (Schraffenberger 2018, 702–705).

38. d   Medicare provides for additional payment for other factors related to a particular hospital's business. If the hospital treats a high percentage of low-income patients, it receives a percentage add-on payment applied to the MS-DRG adjusted base payment rate. This add-on payment, known as the disproportionate share hospital (DSH) adjustment, provides for a percentage increase in Medicare payments to hospitals that qualify under either of two statutory formulas designed to identify hospitals that serve these areas. Hospitals that have approved teaching hospitals also receive a percentage add-on payment for each Medicare discharge paid under IPPS, known as the indirect medical education (IME) adjustment. The percentage varies, depending on the ratio of residents to beds. Additional payments are made for new technologies or medical services that have been approved for special add-on payments. Finally, the costs incurred by a hospital for a Medicare beneficiary are evaluated to determine whether the hospital is eligible for an additional payment as an outlier case. This additional payment is designed to protect the hospital from large financial losses due to unusually expensive cases (Schraffenberger 2018, 702–707).

39. b   Congress directed HHS to conduct a three-year demonstration project using RACs to detect and correct improper payments in the Medicare traditional fee-for-service program. Congress further required HHS to make the RAC program permanent and nationwide by January 1, 2010 (Schraffenberger 2018, 712–714).

40. a   The revenue cycle middle process includes case management, charge capture, clinical documentation review, and coding (Malmgren and Solberg 2016, 246–256).

41. b   Attending and consulting physicians have no bearing on the assignment of the MS-DRG and payment to the hospital (Schraffenberger 2018, 90–91).

42. b   As of January 1, 2011, CMS allows a total of 25 ICD-10-CM diagnosis codes (1 principal and 24 additional diagnoses) for 837 Institutional claims filing (Schraffenberger 2018, 93).

43. b   Billing for two services that are prohibited from being billed on the same day (Amatayakul 2016, 289–292).

44. c   Remittance advice (RA) is sent to the provider to explain payments made by third-party payers (Smith 2019, 305–308).

45. b   The monies collected from third-party payers cannot be greater than the amount of the provider's charges (Hazelwood and Venable 2016, 223–225).

46. c   Improve documentation to support services billed (Sayles and Gordon 2016, 665).

47. c   To qualify for a cost outlier, a hospital's charges for a case (adjusted to cost) must exceed the payment rate for the MS-DRG by a specific threshold amount determined by CMS for each fiscal year (Hazelwood and Venable 2016, 225).

48. c   A *chargemaster* is a financial management form that contains information about the organization's charges for the healthcare services it provides to patients (Gordon and Gordon 2016, 424, 426).

49. a   A *fee schedule* is a list of healthcare services and procedures and charges associated with each (Gordon and Gordon 2016, 427, 442).

50. b   The charge description master includes the charge code, charge code description, CPT/HCPCS code and modifier; revenue code and price (Malmgren and Solberg 2016, 251).

51. a   An advance beneficiary notice (ABN) must be given to the patient to sign before treatment if any indication presents that may cause the service to be denied by Medicare (Hazelwood and Venable 2016, 235–236; Palkie 2016, 295).

52. a   When a physician accepts assignment of benefits, the physician can only collect any applicable deductible or coinsurance from the patient (Casto and Forrestal 2015, 154).

53. c   Budget neutrality must be maintained annually when the RVUs are adjusted (Casto and Forrestal 2015, 154).

54. b   Generally, reimbursement for healthcare services is dependent on patients having health insurance (Casto and Forrestal 2015, 5).

55. a   Health insurance for spouses, children, or both is known as dependent (family) coverage (Casto and Forrestal 2015, 7).

56. b   A complete medical history documents the patient's current complaints and symptoms and lists his or her past medical, personal, and family history (Smith 2018, 220–221, 224).

57. a   *Present on admission* is defined as present at the time the order for inpatient admission occurs (CMS 2018a, Appendix I).

58. b   *Medical history* documents the patient's current complaints and symptoms and lists the patient's past medical, personal, and family history. The physical examination report represents the attending physician's assessment of the patient's current health status (Smith 2019, 235).

59. a   An *operative report* describes the surgical procedures performed on the patient (Brickner 2016, 95).

60. a   All patients meeting the United Network of Organ Sharing criteria must be evaluated with the documentation part of the health record per CMS and the Joint Commission (Reynolds and Sharp, 114).

61. c   A *pathology report* usually includes descriptions of the tissue from a gross or macroscopic level and representative cells at the microscopic level along with interpretive findings (Brickner 2016, 95).

62. c   The American College of Surgeons started its Hospital Standardization Program in 1918 (Sayles 2016, 4).

63. c   All entries must be legible and complete and must be authenticated and dated promptly by the person (identified by name and discipline) who is responsible for ordering, providing, or evaluating the service furnished (42 CFR 482.24).

64. d   In a paper-based health record environment, when corrections are made to health record entries, it is appropriate to draw a single line through the original entry, write "error" above the entry, and then sign the correction, including the date and time (Sayles and Gordon 2016, 65, 70, 127, 204).

65. b   The Accreditation Association for Ambulatory Health Care (AAAHC) has requirements for the content of the ambulatory care record that are provided to ambulatory surgery centers, community health centers, health plans and medical homes and office-based surgery centers (Reynolds and Sharp 2016, 117).

66. c   An addendum may be included in the medical record to update or supplement documentation that has been recorded (Sayles 2016, 65, 69).

67. b   Documentation policies are used to define the acceptable practices that should be followed by all applicable staff to ensure consistency, continuity, and clarity in documentation (Brickner 2016, 82–87).

68. d   In order to thoughtfully and appropriately manage copy functionality, organizations must have sound documentation integrity policies within their organization. HIM professionals should lead their organizations in developing copy policies and procedures that address operational processes, utilization of copy functionality, documentation guidelines, responsibility, and auditing and reporting (AHIMA 2016, 7; Sayles and Gordon, 73, 243, 615–616). Documentation policies are used to define the acceptable practices that should be followed by all applicable staff to ensure consistency and continuity and clarity in documentation (AHIMA 2005; Brinda 2016, 156; Amatayakul 2016, 294).

69. a   The physician principally responsible for the patient's hospital care writes and signs the discharge summary (Fahrenholz and Russo 2013, 284).

70. a   *Histology* refers to the tissue type of a lesion. The histology of tissue is determined by a pathologist and documented in the pathology report (Schraffenberger 2018, 145).

71. a   HIM ethical obligations apply regardless of employment site (Gordon and Gordon 2016b, 612–619).

72. a   *Privacy* is the right of an individual to be left alone (Rinehart-Thompson 2016b, 214; Gordon and Gordon 2016b, 610).

73. a   Corrective action should be taken when error or accuracy rates are deemed to be at an unacceptable rate (Rinehart-Thompson 2016b, 243; Foltz et al. 2016, 459, 461).

74. d   *Standards* are fixed rules that must be followed, which is different from a guideline that provides general direction (Sayles 2016, 66; Brickner 2016, 82).

75. c   Healthcare organizations should have a coding compliance plan in addition to the organization's compliance plan, with the same components (Foltz et al. 2016, 461).

76. d   The addendum must have a separate signature, date, and time from the original entry (Sayles 2016, 65, 69; Brickner 2016, 88; Rinehart-Thompson 2016c, 204).

77. a   An individual's right extends for as long as the record is maintained (Rinehart-Thompson 2016b, 218).

78. c   HIPAA regulations preempt less strict state statutes where they exist (Rinehart-Thompson 2016a, 271).

79. a   The Privacy Rule is applicable to all covered entities involved, either directly or indirectly, with transmitting or performing any electronic transactions specified in the act (Rinehart-Thompson 2016b, 218).

80. d   Confidentiality is the responsibility for limiting disclosure (Rinehart-Thompson 2016b, 214; Gordon and Gordon 2016b, 610).

81. a   The Joint Commission, Commission on Accreditation of Rehabilitation Facilities, and the National Committee for Quality Assurance are all acceptable accrediting bodies for behavioral healthcare settings (Fahrenholz and Russo 2013, 624).

82. b   Each time the patient visits the facility, the same *health/medical record number* is used, allowing communication between past and present healthcare providers and consistent sharing of information regarding the course of treatment (Fahrenholz and Russo 2013, 189).

83. c   State licensure agencies have regulations that are modeled after the Medicare Conditions of Participation and Joint Commission standards. States conduct annual surveys to determine the hospital's continued compliance with licensure standards (Fahrenholz and Russo 2013, 447).

84. b   A *blanket authorization* is a common ethical problem when misused. Patients often sign a blanket authorization, which authorizes the release of information from that point forward, without understanding the implications. The problem is the patient is not aware of what information is being accessed (Gordon and Gordon 2016b, 616).

85. b   Automatic session termination will help to control access to the computer when unattended by automatically ending the session when not in use, preventing unauthorized access (HHS 2006, 4; Rinehart-Thompson 2016a, 264–265).

86. c   Edit checks help ensure data integrity by allowing only reasonable and predetermined values to be entered into the computer (Rinehart-Thompson 2016a, 265).

87. b When several people enter data in an EHR, you can define how users must enter data in specific fields to help maintain consistency. For example, an input mask for a form means that users can only enter the date in a specified format (MacDonald 2010, chapter 4; Carter and Palmer 2016, 506).

88. c Automated systems for registering patients and tracking their encounters are commonly known as registration admission-discharge-transfer (ADT) systems (Amatayakul 2016, 289).

89. b A *data warehouse* is a special type of database that consolidates and stores data from various databases (Oachs and Watters 2016, 998).

90. b The R-ADT systems in hospitals register inpatient and outpatient admissions; captures the demographics and insurance data; and supplies it to the other systems (Amatayakul 2016, 289).

91. a An *encoder* is computer software that helps the coding professional assign codes (Sayles 2016, 75; Amatayakul 2016, 291).

92. c *Natural-language processing* (NLP) uses artificial intelligence software to allow digital text from online documents stored in the organization's information system to be read directly by the software, which then suggests codes to match the documentation (Sayles 2016, 69; Amatayakul 2016, 293; Giannangelo 2016, 326; Foltz et al. 2016, 462).

93. d Regardless of state laws, every person or organization is subject to HIPAA and must comply with it. The law supercedes state law (Rinehart-Thompson 2016b, 217).

94. b *Beneficence* means promoting good (Gordon and Gordon 2016b, 604, 618).

95. d Regardless of state laws, every person or organization is subject to HIPAA and must comply with it. The law supersedes state law (Rinehart-Thompson 2016b, 217).

96. d The distinction of psychotherapy notes is important due to HIPAA requirements that these notes may not be released unless specifically specified in an authorization (Fahrenholz and Russo 2013, 616–617).

97. d When a person or entity willfully and knowingly violates the HIPAA Privacy Rule, a fine of not more than $250,000, not more than 10 years in jail, or both may be imposed (Brinda and Watters 2016, 307–312).

98. d *Access control* means being able to identify which employees should have access to what data (Rinehart-Thompson 2016b, 262–263, 273).

99. b An EHR can be viewed by multiple users and from multiple locations at any time, and organizations must have in place appropriate security access control measures to ensure the safety of the data (Sayles 2016, 53; Amatayakul 2016, 285; Kellogg 2016b, 482–483).

100. c When a state law is more stringent than a federal law, hospitals must comply with both (Fahrenholz and Russo 2013, 436).

REFERENCES

42 CFR 482.24: Medical Record Services. 2010.

Amatayakul, M. K. 2016. Health Information Technologies. Chapter 11 in *Health Information Management Technology: An Applied Approach*, 5th ed. Edited by N. B. Sayles and L. L. Gordon. Chicago: AHIMA.

American Health Information Management Association (AHIMA). 2018. *Clinical Coding Workout: Practice Exercises for Skill Development with Answers*. 2018 ed. Chicago: AHIMA.

American Health Information Management Association (AHIMA). 2016 update. *Copy Functionality Toolkit*. Chicago: AHIMA.

American Health Information Management Association (AHIMA). 2011. e-HIM Work Group on Maintaining the Legal EHR. Update: Maintaining a legally sound health record—Paper and electronic. *Journal of AHIMA* 76(10):64A–L. Chicago: AHIMA.

American Medical Association. 2018. *CPT Current Procedural Terminology Professional Edition*. Chicago: AMA.

American Medical Association. 1994–2010. *CPT Current Procedural Terminology Changes: An Insider's View*. Chicago: AMA.

Brickner, M. R. 2016. Health Record Content and Documentation. Chapter 4 in *Health Information Management Technology: An Applied Approach*, 5th ed. Edited by N. B. Sayles and L. L. Gordon. Chicago: AHIMA.

Brinda, D. 2016. Data Management. Chapter 6 in *Health Information Management Technology: An Applied Approach*, 5th ed. Edited by N. B. Sayles and L. L. Gordon. Chicago: AHIMA.

Brinda, D. and A. Watters. 2016. Data Privacy, Confidentiality, and Security. Chapter 11 in *Health Information Management: Concepts, Principles, and Practice* 5th ed. Edited by P. Oachs and A. Watters. Chicago: AHIMA.

Brodnik, M., L. Rinehart-Thompson, and R. Reynolds. 2016. *Fundamentals of Law for Health Informatics and Information Management*, 3rd ed. Revised Reprint. Chicago: AHIMA.

Carter, D. and M. N. Palmer. 2016. Performance Improvement. Chapter 18 in *Health Information Management Technology: An Applied Approach*, 5th ed. Edited by N. B. Sayles and L. L. Gordon. Chicago: AHIMA.

Casto, A. 2018. *Principles of Healthcare Reimbursement*, 6th ed. Chicago: AHIMA.

Centers for Medicare and Medicaid Services (CMS). 2018a. ICD-10-CM Official Guidelines for Coding and Reporting. http://www.cdc.gov/nchs/data/icd/10cmguidelines_2017_final.pdf.

Centers for Medicare and Medicaid Services (CMS). 2018b. Official ICD-10-PCS Coding Guidelines. https://www.cms.gov/Medicare/Coding/ICD10/Downloads/2017-Official-ICD-10-PCS-Coding -Guidelines.pdf.

Centers for Medicare and Medicaid Services (CMS). 2018c. National Correct Coding Initiative Policy Manual for Medicare Services. https://www.cms.gov/Medicare/Coding/NationalCorrectCodInitEd /Downloads/2018-NCCI-Policy-Manual.zip.

Centers for Medicare and Medicaid Services (CMS). 2017. ICD-10-PCS Reference Manual. https:// www.cms.gov/Medicare/Coding/ICD10/2017-ICD-10-PCS-and-GEMs.html.

Department of Health and Human Services (HHS). 2006. HIPAA Security Guidance. http://www.hhs .gov/sites/default/files/ocr/privacy/hipaa/administrative/securityrule/remoteuse.pdf.

Fahrenholz, C. G. 2016. *Documentation for Health Records*, 2nd ed. Chicago: AHIMA.

Foltz, D. A., K. M. Lankisch, and N. B. Sayles. 2016. Fraud and Abuse Compliance. Chapter 16 in *Health Information Management Technology: An Applied Approach*, 5th ed. Edited by N. B. Sayles and L. L. Gordon. Chicago: AHIMA.

Gordon, L. L. and M. L. Gordon. 2016a. Revenue Management and Reimbursement. Chapter 15 in *Health Information Management Technology: An Applied Approach*, 5th ed. Edited by N. B. Sayles and L. L. Gordon. Chicago: AHIMA.

Gordon, L. L. and M. L. Gordon. 2016b. Management. Chapter 19 in *Health Information Management Technology: An Applied Approach*, 5th ed. Edited by N. B. Sayles and L. L. Gordon. Chicago: AHIMA.

Hazelwood, A. C. and C. A. Venable. 2016. Reimbursement Methodologies. Chapter 7 in *Health Information Management: Concepts, Principles, and Practice* 5th ed. Edited by P. Oachs and A. Watters. Chicago: AHIMA.

Hazelwood, A. and C. Venable. 2014. *Diagnostic Coding for Physician Services: ICD-10-CM*. 2014 ed. Chicago: AHIMA.

Horton, L. A. 2016. Healthcare Statistics. Chapter 14 in *Health Information Management Technology: An Applied Approach*, 5th ed. Edited by N. B. Sayles and L. L. Gordon. Chicago: AHIMA.

Kellogg, D. W. 2016a. Healthcare Delivery Systems. Chapter 2 in *Health Information Management Technology: An Applied Approach*, 5th ed. Edited by N. B. Sayles and L. L. Gordon. Chicago: AHIMA.

Kellogg, D. W. 2016b. Leadership. Chapter 17 in *Health Information Management Technology: An Applied Approach*, 5th ed. Edited by N. B. Sayles and L. L. Gordon. Chicago: AHIMA.

Kuehn, L. 2019. *Procedural Coding and Reimbursement for Physician Services: Applying Current Procedural Terminology and HCPCS*. Chicago: AHIMA.

Kuehn, L. and T. Jorwic. 2018. *ICD-10-PCS: An Applied Approach*. Chicago: AHIMA.

MacDonald, M. 2010. *Access 2010: The Missing Manual*. Sebastopol, CA: O'Reilly Media, Inc.

Malmgren, C. and C. J. Solberg. 2016. Revenue Cycle Management. Chapter 8 in *Health Information Management: Concepts, Principles, and Practice* 5th ed. Edited by P. Oachs and A. Watters. Chicago: AHIMA.

Oachs, P. and A. Watters, eds. 2016. *Health Information Management: Concepts, Principles, and Practice*. 5th ed. Chicago: AHIMA.

O'Dell, R. M. 2016. Clinical Quality Management. Chapter 21 in *Health Information Management: Concepts, Principles, and Practice* 5th ed. Edited by P. Oachs and A. Watters. Chicago: AHIMA.

Palkie, B. 2016. Clinical Classifications, Vocabularies, Terminologies, and Standards. Chapter 5 in *Health Information Management: Concepts, Principles, and Practice* 5th ed. Edited by P. Oachs and A. Watters. Chicago: AHIMA.

Prater, V. S. 2016. Human Resources Management and Professional Development. Chapter 20 in *Health Information Management Technology: An Applied Approach*, 5th ed. Edited by N. B. Sayles and L. L. Gordon. Chicago: AHIMA.

Reynolds, R. B. and M. Sharp. 2016. Health Record Content and Documentation. Chapter 4 in *Health Information Management: Concepts, Principles, and Practice* 5th ed. Edited by P. Oachs and A. Watters. Chicago: AHIMA.

Rinehart-Thompson, L. A. 2016a. Data Security. Chapter 10 in *Health Information Management Technology: An Applied Approach*, 5th ed. Edited by N. B. Sayles and L. L. Gordon. Chicago: AHIMA.

Rinehart-Thompson, L. A. 2016b. Data Privacy and Confidentiality. Chapter 9 in *Health Information Management Technology: An Applied Approach*, 5th ed. Edited by N. B. Sayles and L. L. Gordon. Chicago: AHIMA.

Rinehart-Thompson, L. A. 2016c. Health Law. Chapter 8 in *Health Information Management Technology: An Applied Approach*, 5th ed. Edited by N. B. Sayles and L. L. Gordon. Chicago: AHIMA.

Russo, R. 2010. *Clinical Documentation Improvement: Achieving Excellence*. Chicago: AHIMA.

Sandefer, R. H. 2016. Health Information Technologies. Chapter 12 in *Health Information Management: Concepts, Principles, and Practice* 5th ed. Edited by P. Oachs and A. Watters. Chicago: AHIMA.

Sayles, N. B. 2016. Health Information Functions, Purpose, and Users. Chapter 3 in *Health Information Management Technology: An Applied Approach*, 5th ed. Edited by N. B. Sayles and L. L. Gordon. Chicago: AHIMA.

Sayles, N. and K. Trawick. 2014. *Introduction to Computer Systems for Health Information Technology*, 2nd ed. Chicago: AHIMA.

Schraffenberger, L.A. 2019. *Basic ICD-10-CM and ICD-10-PCS Coding*. Chicago: AHIMA.

Smith, G. 2019. *Basic Current Procedural Terminology and HCPCS Coding*. Chicago: AHIMA.